To Brook

Seize Each Day

THE MAN WHO LOST HIMSELF

Terry Evanshen

THE MAN WHO LOST HIMSELF

THE TERRY EVANSHEN STORY

JUNE CALLWOOD

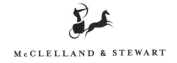

McCLELLAND & STEWART

Canadian Cataloguing in Publication Data

Callwood, June
    The man who lost himself: the Terry Evanshen story

ISBN 978-0-7710-1863-3 (bound)
ISBN 978-0-7710-1864-9 (pbk.)

1. Evanshen, Terry, 1944-   – Health. 2. Brain damage – patients – Canada – Biography. 3. Motivational speakers – Canada – Biography. 4. Football players – Canada – Biography. I. Title.

RC387.5.C34 2000   362.1'97481'0092   C00-930073-2

We acknowledge the financial support of the Government of Canada through the Book Publishing Industry Development Program for our publishing activities. We further acknowledge the support of the Canada Council for the Arts and the Ontario Arts Council for our publishing program.

Typeset in Bembo by M&S, Toronto
Printed and bound in Canada

McClelland & Stewart Ltd.
75 Sherbourne Street
Toronto, Ontario
M5A 2P9
www.mcclelland.com

2   3   4   5   10   09   08   07

To the valiant Terry and Lorraine

ONE

At a quarter to six on the evening of Monday, July 4, 1988, in the final moments of his first life, Terry Evanshen was speaking on his car phone to his youngest daughter, eleven-year-old Jennifer. His family was waiting for him to start the barbecue for steaks, and he wanted them to know he was only a few minutes away from home.

If Terry had been counting his blessings in the seconds that remained to him, he would have experienced a flash of intense contentment which the great Brandeis psychologist Abraham Maslow called a "peak experience," an epiphany of sublime inner harmony.

For a start, it was a jewel of a summer day, with the sun still high in a cloudless sky and a breeze that promised an end to the weekend's heat wave. Terry was driving his new vehicle, a silver-grey Jeep Cherokee, a possession that delighted him. All the windows were up and the air conditioner was at full blast. To the dismay of his family, that was just the way he liked it. Two days earlier he had completed a successful three-week jaunt around Europe selling small ceramic room heaters, a Canadian invention that he estimated would make him over a hundred thousand dollars in commissions, maybe two. He had just passed his forty-fourth birthday, and, a non-smoker who exercised regularly and rarely drank, he was in extraordinarily fine physical condition, with the hard muscular body of his athletic youth. Waiting for him near Brooklin, a village northeast of Toronto, was his heritage stone farmhouse on thirty-two acres of rolling countryside, with a newly installed swimming pool and riding horses in the barn. Lorraine, his spunky wife of twenty-two years, would have a welcoming quip, and their three beautiful, smart daughters would come running for hugs.

Terry might also have reflected in that good moment on his past glories. He was wearing the evidence, a bulky gold ring that indicated he had played on a Grey Cup champion team in the Canadian Football League. For fourteen years, from 1965 to 1978, he had been a professional football player. At slightly under five foot ten, he was one of the smallest men in the league, but he was an indomitable and gutsy wide receiver with an astonishing lifetime record of only three fumbles. He scored two touchdowns in the 1968 Grey Cup final that his team, the Calgary Stampeders, lost, but he was a star with the 1970 Montreal Alouettes when they won the Cup. Then there was his induction into the Canadian Football Hall of Fame; at forty, he was the youngest player ever to be so honoured.

Ahead of him as Terry drove west along Winchester Road was the intersection at Simcoe Street. Both roads are well-travelled arteries that meet in flat farmland just north of Oshawa. Three of the corners at the crossing are owned by Windfields Farm, the fabled thoroughbred stable that produced the great stallion Northern Dancer, and those corners are marked by the distinctive rail fencing of a horse spread. The fourth corner is tilled land, the owner's prosperous house visible far up the road.

The light for east-west traffic on Winchester was green. As Terry drove his Jeep across the intersection at moderate speed, a 1981 blue GMC van, a Chevy, came at him from his left. It was travelling north on Simcoe at a good clip and ran the red light. The Chevy slammed into the middle of the Jeep at a right angle, a collision which police and ambulance crews call a T-bone. The impact rotated the Jeep in a flat spin and then something tipped it and it flew into the air, turning end over end.

That's what Debbie Parry saw. She was driving east on Winchester on her way home from work with two passengers in her car, both of them from her office. She remembers that the east-west traffic light was green, so she slowed but did not stop before turning right onto Simcoe, going south towards Oshawa. Just after she made the turn, she heard the sickening sound of crashing metal. Looking in her rear-view mirror, she saw a vehicle flying through the air. The Jeep slammed down hard on its wheels on the road, making a deep gouge in the pavement, and then rolled over once on the slope of the shoulder. It came to a lurching stop upright on cockeyed wheels amid a litter of crumbled metal and broken glass, its left side bowed inward.

Terry was no longer inside. The force of the van's crash into the Jeep's driver's door had ripped his seat belt from its mooring and blasted him the length of the Jeep and out the rear window. Terry landed on his face in mown weeds about fifteen feet behind his vehicle.

A ghastly silence fell.

The first people to move were those in the line of cars facing south on Simcoe Street and stopped for the red light. Shelagh Donaldson, now Shelagh Pulo, was driving the third of the cars waiting for the light to change. Nineteen years old, Shelagh was on her way to Oshawa and a new job as night security guard at a trucking company. She didn't see the crash, but she heard it and saw the Jeep in a flat spin, followed by a shocking flip in the air.

She thought, "Oh, my God," and then she was out of her car, running to the crushed vehicle. She reached it at the same time as Glen Maughan, twenty-six, driver of a truck stopped three cars behind her. A carpenter, Maughan was driving home from a job renovating a kitchen. When the crash occurred, he was lighting a cigarette, his head down, but he heard the "horrendous" noise of metal over the sound of his turned-up stereo. He looked up and was appalled to see the Jeep high in the air to his right. He watched, frozen, as it hit the road and rolled.

Maughan leaped out of his car and joined Shelagh Donaldson, who was peering in the driver's side of the Jeep. They were amazed to find the seat empty. Mystified, they ran around to the back, where they could smell gasoline and hear fluid pouring from the ruptured fuel tank. Some distance from the car they found a barefoot man dressed in a shredded T-shirt and casual pants, lying prone in the weeds with his head turned to one side. His body looked battered, with dozens of small cuts starting to bleed, and multiple pieces of glass glittering in his left arm. He seemed to be sleeping peacefully.

Maughan was aghast to see blood trickling from the man's ear. He stooped and put his hand under the man's nose and was reassured to feel breath.

Donaldson was newly graduated from a community college course in corrections (prison and security work). Her training had included cardiopulmonary resuscitation (CPR) and first aid. Crouched by the inert man, she hoped fervently that she would not be required to practise either. She said later, "I was so relieved that he was breathing. I didn't want to have to do something and maybe get it wrong."

She stood up and looked at the horrified motorists gathering around the prone man. She was puzzled that they were staring expectantly at her. She realized that she was wearing her security guard uniform, which somehow had conveyed the impression that she would know what to do. Though her heart was pounding, she went along with their assumption, and moved into the authority vacuum. She warned bystanders about the gasoline-soaked ground, and picked at random two people whom she asked to direct traffic around the scene. Meanwhile, the driver of the Chevy who had run the red light was out of his van, wandering around in a confused state with blood streaming down his face.

The last thing Donaldson wanted to do was move the unconscious man, despite the foreboding fumes of gasoline and the danger of fire. She had been taught that inept handling of an injured person can cause paralysis if there is damage to the spinal cord. She checked anxiously, but the man was still breathing. Maughan, whose first-aid training was with St. John's Ambulance, was thinking the same: *let's not touch him.*

Donaldson remembers, "The man looked about twenty years old, about my age, and I thought, 'You poor guy.' I figured he had to be badly hurt, given what his body had gone through, and I was sorry for him because he was so young."

The most immediate concern was the seeping gasoline, particularly as the weeds in which Terry lay were tinder-dry. A double line of hydro towers marches across the intersection, and Donaldson believed that the Trans-Canada Pipeline was under them, buried right beneath her feet. In her excited state, she was thinking *explosion*. She asked the gathering crowd if anyone had a fire extinguisher in their car. They shook their heads.

While Donaldson worried about the spilled gasoline, others were trying to decide the quickest way to summon help. In 1988, cell phones were a novelty and no one had one. A third vehicle had been involved in the collision, another blue van. It was the first vehicle in the line of southbound traffic waiting at the red light. The Chevy van that hit the Jeep had been travelling at such speed that even though its front end was demolished it continued through the intersection and smashed into the stopped van. The driver of the second van, James Irvine, was bleeding from his nose and cradling a sore arm, but he volunteered to telephone. The garage where he worked was less than two minutes away, he said. Someone offered to drive him and they roared away, but they had been gone only seconds when a truck stopped at the scene and the driver used his two-way radio to sound the alarm.

Much as she was loath to disturb the unconscious man, Donaldson was close to panic at the danger of fire. She had just made the decision to carry him a safe distance from the Jeep when someone hurried up with a fire extinguisher. Seconds later an ambulance arrived.

The call for help had been relayed to fire and ambulance dispatchers and to the Durham Police Force. The police staff sergeant who answered the phone looked around the parade room and his eye fell on a rookie, Constable Charles Nash, known as Chuck, twenty-one years old, fresh out of police college and with only two weeks' experience of patrolling solo. Nash, a gangly six foot two and strikingly handsome, has an endearing quality of earnest decency. "Nash," the staff sergeant said. "There's an accident with an injury, and you're doing it." As Nash picked up his hat and headed for the door, the sergeant offered some kindly advice.

"Don't fuck it up," he said.

By extraordinary good fortune, the ambulance paramedics who received the call from the dispatcher were only blocks from the scene. Jim Jack and Craig Jones, at that time among the most competent paramedics in the country, happened to be cruising nearby because they had decided to stop for some Baskin Robbins ice cream before reporting to base at the Oshawa General Hospital to start their night shift.

Jones was driving. As allowed in a Code Four, the ambulance designation for life-and-death emergencies, he hit the siren and headed at top speed for Simcoe and Winchester. Jack checked his kit to make sure it contained the essentials for responding to serious trauma and it crossed his mind that they were answering yet another "blue-sky" accident. Ambulance crews find it strange that they see their most horrible motor accident injuries when the weather is fine. They assume that drivers slow down for a sleet storm, thus reducing the impact of any collision, and speed when there is good visibility and dry pavement. Still, it strikes paramedics as odd.

When the ambulance came to a hard-brake stop at the scene, the paramedics split up without consultation, each of them familiar with the drill. Both made a quick survey and assessment of the scene. Responsibility for tending the most injured person fell to Jim Jack. With his kit in one hand and an oxygen tank in the other, he hurried to the man on the ground. Jones, as driver, had the job of caring for the next-most injured person, making the decision about calling for another ambulance — which he did, promptly — and studying the wrecked vehicles in order to reconstruct how the injuries happened. This is critical information for the staff in hospital emergency rooms, who need to know, for instance, if the steering wheel was involved, in which case chest damage can be expected, or if there was contact with the windshield, which would set up another array of possibilities, and what metal at what force whacked the patient's body. So routine is the requirement to assess wreckage that paramedics do this on automatic pilot, without pausing in the primary task of helping the wounded.

Jones went to the driver of the Chevy van who had caused the collision, Daryl Pertan, thirty-seven, a bearded, long-haired, self-employed contractor who had been hurrying home from work. He was bleeding so heavily from deep gashes in his scalp that his eye sockets were full of blood and he could scarcely see. Someone asked him, "What the hell happened?" He mumbled, "I wish I knew." The paramedic pulled on latex gloves, sat Pertan down, and started to work on the cuts.

While Jones was tending to Pertan, Jack was inspecting Terry Evanshen's limp body. He was alarmed to see that the man's skin was a dusky blue, "as blue as jeans." Terry was still breathing, though shallowly, but for some reason his blood wasn't getting oxygen. In a few minutes he would be dead from asphyxiation, but there was still a pulse, and maybe he could be saved.

Terry later came to believe that he stopped breathing for four minutes, something the family was told in the hospital, and that a paramedic revived him. Jack says no. "When you're dead from trauma," he explains bluntly, "you stay dead." He doesn't mean that paramedics don't try to resuscitate an injured person who has stopped breathing, but only that ninety-nine percent of the time the effort is futile.

Resuscitation attempts have a better outcome when the victim has had a heart attack or was drowning. In those cases, paramedics, lifeguards and others in front-line rescue work are usually successful in efforts to revive a person who isn't breathing. Modern techniques make it possible to restart a heart, pump oxygen into lungs, and restore vital signs to a person who seems dead. Jack says that once he was part of a team who restarted the heart of a man who was electrocuted when he hit a TV antenna and fell off a tall ladder. He had no pulse when they got to him, but they got his heart pumping again and he walked out of the hospital feeling just fine. He lived because it was the electric shock that had stopped his breathing, not the fall.

It's a tough call if rescuers don't know how long the victim has been without oxygen. Depending on how long breathing is stopped – ten minutes is the far outside edge of the envelope – and a myriad other factors, people may be revived, but the long oxygen deprivation can cause so much brain damage that they remain forever in a coma, living corpses attached to machines and beyond the reach of communication.

As Jim Jack opened his kit he examined the circle of people standing around him. Picking a man who looked composed, he said, "Come here. I need you to hold his head. If he starts to come around, don't let his head move." Jack watched until he saw that the man understood the instruction, and then got to work.

Terry Evanshen was getting the help of a top-of-the-line paramedic. Thirty-three years old, Jim Jack, a big man with a full beard and long hair, had graduated only four years earlier as an ambulance attendant, but he was a keener, and he was working with an ambulance service that had decided to make itself the best anywhere. That attitude can happen in small centres, and Oshawa is a tough, bustling, lunch-bucket city that relies on the auto industry and on its own combative spirit. Oshawa paramedics were so dedicated to upgrading their skills, even though they received no extra pay for it, that they set the provincial standard and were rated the best paramedics in Ontario. Once a year in the 1980s they competed with ambulance teams in the United States, comporting themselves handily.

"The service was full of bright people at that time," Jack says. "We had a lot of pride in our history, and we were proud of what we could do."

The first rule of a paramedic or a hospital emergency team is the same: secure the airway. Jack needed to roll Terry over to determine what was blocking his oxygen intake, but the procedure is dangerous when there is a possibility of a spinal cord injury. At that moment help arrived. A second ambulance pulled up nearby and Andy Benson, the driver, leaped out. Benson took the bystander's place at Terry's head and got set. "Let's turn 'im," Jack said tersely.

What happened next is one of the most critical manoeuvres in life-saving. If injured people have a high fracture of the spine, careless handling can cause quadriplegia. Andy Benson knelt, crossed his arms and put his hands firmly on either side of Terry's head. Jim Jack grasped Terry's left shoulder and hip. On a count, he rolled Terry over on his back while Benson held his head steadily in line with the spine and extended from the shoulders, ending the movement with his hands uncrossed. Paramedics practice this deft exercise over and over. And over.

"It doesn't do to save a man's life and make him paralysed," Jack comments dryly.

Fire trucks arrived, and Jack stopped worrying about the stench of gasoline. Right behind them was Constable Chuck Nash in a yellow Durham Police Force cruiser. Nash had been drifting north on Simcoe Street at a reasonable speed when the fire trucks passed him. "Uh-oh," he thought. "Better step on it." To his chagrin, two ambulances and two fire department vehicles were at the accident ahead of him, and his was the last emergency-response vehicle to arrive. Traffic was partially blocked in all four directions and dozens of people were milling about in the middle of the intersection as though it were a pedestrian mall. As Nash took in the magnitude of his assignment, his heart sank. For an instant he had a craven wish to change into civilian clothes and disappear into the crowd, but that flare of dread passed. Stolidly, he made a note of the time of his arrival, five minutes after six, and climbed out of the cruiser.

He had the scene-of-accident check list in his head: *Attend to the injured.* Four paramedics were doing that. *Preserve evidence.* He had to make sure the bystanders didn't disturb the debris on the road, making it more difficult for experts to reconstruct what had happened. *Should the road be closed?* Yes, he decided. He radioed for assistance. Both highways, as it turned out, would be blocked off for hours. *Make certain bystanders are safe.* Until other cruisers arrived, he would warn people to get out of the way of any car attempting to thread the intersection. *Redirect traffic.* An off-duty police officer said she would take care of that until reinforcements came. *Are the traffic lights in working order?* Yes. *Interview witnesses.* Nash pulled out his notebook.

Jim Jack was checking inside Terry's mouth. A swallowed tongue could account for the cyanotic blueness of the unconscious man's skin, but Terry's tongue was where it was supposed to be. Jack would have continued to look for a blocked airway, but he remembered his glimpse of the Jeep, and the smashed left side where the driver had been sitting. On a hunch that the impact had crushed the man's left chest, Jack opened Terry's shirt. Paramedics frequently have to do this to find the source of a problem, but it can be a tricky matter when the injured person is a woman. With the inevitable curious crowd pressing close, issues of modesty arise to complicate the decision.

As Terry's shirt fell away, the reason for his blueness became painfully obvious. When people breathe, both sides of the chest move together, but Terry's chest was moving out of sync. The left chest wall was falling as the right chest wall rose. He had a flailed chest, an injury most commonly found when the driver's body has smashed into the steering wheel. Several of the ribs on Terry's left side were in loose pieces in his chest.

"Bad trouble," thought Jack. The injured man could take in air, but he couldn't exhale because the floating ribs could not brace the lung to assist it to empty. And because Terry couldn't push air out, there was little lung space for oxygenated air to flow in. Terry was dying of hypoxia – lack of oxygen – exactly as if he were drowning in six feet of water.

Jack pressed his hand hard on the fluttering diaphragm to provide compression, and felt a bubble-wrap crackling under his hand, an indication that air was infiltrating the chest. The left lung must be torn.

Meanwhile, Craig Jones had turned over the two other injured drivers to the second ambulance crew, and ran to assist Jack, who was checking Terry's vital signs. His pulse rate was ninety-six, which was on the high side, but not in itself a worry. When people perceive themselves to be in danger, the body's primitive response is a rush of adrenalin that signals the heart to pump increased blood to the muscles in preparation for the flight-or-fight response. Terry's heartbeat was strong, which suggested that the organ was intact. His respiratory rate was twenty-eight: fast, but not a worry. Skin condition was dry, which is a better status than sweaty skin, a sign of shock. Blood was seeping from the left ear: not good. His pupils were very tiny, but they matched, which was encouraging. When one pupil is larger than the other, a condition known laconically as a "blown" pupil, it could be evidence of brain damage. Moving rapidly, Jack gave Terry some harmless pain, pinching the big muscle between neck and shoulder. There was no reaction from the inert man, which was not good at all.

He opened Terry's mouth and passed into his throat an airway tube, a stiff plastic pipe with a flange on the top end that would keep the breathing passage open and prevent Terry's tongue from blocking it. Then Jack dug from his kit a non-rebreather oxygen mask. When connected to a portable oxygen tank, the mask delivers pure oxygen. With Jones's help, he clamped the mask over Terry's mouth and nose, and attached the mask to the oxygen tank.

As soon as the flow of oxygen began, a magical transformation occurred. Terry's skin turned from the fatal blueness to a normal colour. The mask, coupled with Jack's pressure on the left diaphragm, was allowing oxygen to get through to Terry's starved blood.

More people were stopping their cars and getting out to look at the carnage. One of them, wandering on the perimeter, picked up what appeared to be a woman's zippered purse. Glen Maughan, the man who, with Shelagh Donaldson, had found Terry, thought, "My God, there was a second person thrown out of the Jeep." He started to look for a woman's body in the long uncut grass along the fenceline.

Jack told Jones to get the backboard and MAST pants from the ambulance. The pants, invented by American medics during the war in Vietnam, were an emergency measure for heavily bleeding soldiers, and for years afterwards were a common accessory in North American ambulances. Rarely used in recent years, they are an inflatable wraparound for the legs and lower torso that fasten with Velcro strips. When inflated, the pants function much like a blood-pressure cuff, cutting off circulation to the lower body in order to maximize the blood supply to the vital organs of heart, lungs, and brain. Compressing blood circulation buys badly injured people transportation time, but the use of MAST pants is so problematic that in peacetime only a doctor can order them inflated. The chancy issues are that they increase blood loss when the upper body is damaged, and deflating them is a treacherous undertaking because dammed-up blood rushes to the lower body with a force that can drop blood pressure drastically. The paramedics were not yet in contact with a doctor, but the pants needed to be ready in case the order was given.

Jack and Jones were working against a clock in their heads. Long experience has shown ambulance crews that a badly injured person has a "golden" hour, and not many minutes more, between the time of the accident and the first surgical intervention at a hospital. After an hour, chances of survival go down.

On his Ambulance Call Report, Jack later put 18:02 as the time he started work on Terry – "only a guess," he admits – and stabilized the flailed segment of chest with hand pressure. The same report shows he inserted the airway tube less than a minute after that and, moments later, Terry was on oxygen. No one was checking a watch, but that time frame is fairly certain, given the high level of Jim Jack's competence. It is impossible to know, however, exactly how long Terry was oxygen-deprived before the paramedics arrived. And that unaccountable time matters, because somewhere in those few minutes when Terry Evanshen's brain was battered and then starved of oxygen, his memory and his sweet capacity to love and laugh emptied as cleanly as water poured from a cup.

Jack's left hand was still holding down the flailed chest, so Jones pulled a two-pound sandbag out of his kit. Jack moved his hand out of the way while Jones taped the bag tightly against Terry's loose ribs. Oshawa paramedics made their sandbags themselves out of intravenous bags and washed sand.

Jones arranged the splayed-open MAST pants on the backboard. He and Jack expertly rolled Terry's inert body on top of them and fastened the Velcro straps, but left the pants deflated. Then they lashed the heavy straps of the backboard tightly around Terry's body to immobilize him. Jack estimated the straps were in place at 18:17.

Jack then fastened a spiral cervical "stiff neck" collar around Terry's neck and placed sandbags on either side to immobilize his head. The men stretched two Elastoplast strips anchored on the sandbags, one across Terry's forehead and the other over his chin. They were ready to roll. Jack and Jones lifted the backboard and slid it onto the stretcher in the ambulance as Andy Benson sprang behind the wheel. Time: 18:20. Not bad. Approximately eighteen minutes to get the man oxygenated and stabilized.

Constable Chuck Nash joined them. Jones caught his eye, made a thumbs-down sign, and shook his head. He said, "This is the worst chest injury I've ever seen."

"Do you know who he is?" Nash asked.

"No," answered Jones. "He's a John Doe." A pat-check of Terry's pants pockets had turned up no identification.

Carrying the purse that had been found near the Jeep, Glen Maughan approached the officer. Worried that a woman was lying injured in the weeds, Nash asked people clustered around him to mount a shoulder-to-shoulder hunt. Shelagh Donaldson had been trained in grid searches as part of her recent college diploma, so she recruited Maughan and others to march through the grass, eyes on the ground, and then wheel around ninety degrees and walk through the same area crossways. "A human rake," Maughan called it. No one was there.

The purse could only belong to the driver. Chuck Nash looked at it more carefully and saw that it was not a woman's purse. It was a leather Daytimer with a zipper closure and several compartments. In a side pocket he found about $200 U.S. in cash, and also a name: Terry Evanshen. Nash radioed his base that John Doe had been identified, and he gave an address. A supervisor would get in touch with the family. By the time Nash called in, a check had been run on Terry's licence plate, confirming both the name and the address.

Benson started the ambulance while Jim Jack crouched next to the comatose man in the rear. As the ambulance pulled away with its siren screaming, Jack slipped an intravenous needle connected to a saline solution into Terry's right forearm. It would compensate for the fluids being lost from internal bleeds. Injured people can lose massive amounts of blood that pools in their chests, bellies, and extremities without any external sign of blood, so Jack used a large-bore needle to get plenty of replacement fluid moving.

What he didn't know was that the IV "went bad." Since Jack was working in a fast-moving, jolting ambulance, the circumstances for inserting the needle were not ideal, and somehow he had missed the vein. Instead the saline solution was going into tissue and Terry's arm was filling with salt water.

To check the heart rate, Jack attached to Terry's chest a cardiac monitor that could be read in the hospital emergency room, and he made another scan of vital signs. There was little improvement, beyond the significant one of the absence of blueness in skin colour. On the Glasgow Coma Score, which measures depth of coma by noting responses to such stimuli as light, voice, and pain, the unconscious man was scoring a three, the lowest measurement on the scale. Below three, the brain probably is dead. Terry's chest movement was still uneven, despite the pressure of the sandbag. On the hopeful side, his skin was still dry, so he wasn't slipping into shock. The coma might even be lifting a little because he had begun to react to pain stimulus with grimaces and twitches.

Pulling his radio from the pouch on his hip, Jack patched in to the Oshawa General Hospital, just down the road on Simcoe Street. It was not only the nearest emergency room but also was superbly staffed, because Oshawa General, known since an amalgamation in 1998 as Lakeridge Health Corporation, was the largest and busiest non-teaching hospital in the province. Jack gave a terse summary of the vital signs and injuries he could see or guess. Did the doctor want the MAST pants inflated? The doctor on duty, Erik Paidra, looked at the vital signs report and the reading from the heart monitor. He made a fast decision: "Don't inflate."

Extensive injuries such as Terry's are treated at the hospital's busy emergency room every two weeks or so. Highway accident victims are scattered among the routine forty thousand fractures, cuts, fevers, strokes, heart attacks, and burns seen every year, but no one ever gets used to the mess that a bad collision can make of the human body. Jack advised that the incoming man had sustained his injuries from an impact at high speed to the driver's door. That meant Paidra might be seeing full-body damage — head, chest, abdomen, brain, and extremities. The emergency team called in a respiratory therapist and braced itself.

In the ambulance, Jack took Terry's vital signs again. They were holding. It was 6:24. The man was still unconscious, so Jack could be almost certain that his brain was injured. This could mean that the buffeted brain was swelling inside the hard cavity of the skull, and sustaining more damage from its confinement.

Until the late 1990s, the procedure to counteract this ballooning was always to hyperventilate the patient. This "blows off" carbon dioxide, and theoretically causes blood vessels to constrict and the brain to stop bloating. Hyperventilation is now controversial, some maintaining that shrinking blood vessels is not a good idea while a brain is struggling to recover, but in 1988 it was the standard response. To hyperventilate Terry, Jack removed the non-rebreather mask and replaced it with a mask whose flow of oxygen he could control by squeezing a bulb, a process known as "bagging." This procedure is not without risk. If there is a tear in the patient's lung or the pleural sac around the lung, the forced air could go where it shouldn't, exacerbating the rupture. But Jack judged that this was no time for timid measures. It meant that both of the paramedic's hands were occupied, the left one holding the mask tightly over Terry's mouth and nose while the right one squeezed the bulb every three seconds, twenty times a minute. The patient didn't stir. Jack was worried. Why was he still unconscious?

The hospital was about five kilometres from the accident scene. By running red lights with the siren on, the ambulance turned in to the driveway to the emergency doors about five minutes after leaving the scene of the accident.

Back at the intersection, Constable Chuck Nash was busy. People gathered around, wanting to tell him that the Jeep was crossing on a green light and the other driver clearly was at fault. He took down names of four witnesses, Shelagh Donaldson, Glen Maughan, Derek Brazier, and Debbie Parry. Though Debbie Parry had avoided approaching the injured man, having no wish to see a torn-up person, she had remained at the scene out of a sense of civic responsibility so that she could tell the police that the Jeep had had the right-of-way. When Nash had the four names in his pristine police notebook, and all of them confirmed that the blue van was running a red light, he talked to the offending driver, who was about to be loaded into the second ambulance.

Without noticing the transition himself, Chuck Nash was no longer an overwhelmed rookie. As he had gone about the tasks he remembered from police college, his calm professionalism had been above reproach, and he was feeling a measure of satisfaction. What he needed to do next was establish if alcohol had been involved in the collision. He questioned Pertan, the driver of the blue van, watching his behaviour, listening for slurring, leaning close to smell his breath. He decided that the man was completely sober, though badly rattled. In answer to the question, "Can you tell me what happened?" Pertan could only shake his head, his expression a mask of bewilderment. He simply had no idea. He said, "All I know is that I was driving along and suddenly there was a bang."

At the hospital, fire and police personnel were arriving to help the paramedics. With Jim Jack still operating the air bag and holding the mask, Andy Benson and a fireman manoeuvred the gurney through the sliding doors of the emergency department, wheeled it sharp left and down three doors to a miniature operating room, OR4, where major trauma victims are taken for surgery-related emergency procedures.

Under the glare of overhead lights in the hospital corridor, Benson noticed a massive gold ring on the inert man's right hand, and thought, *That looks like a Super Bowl ring.* He bent to examine it closer and recognized the insignia of the Canadian Football League. A football fan, he was awed. He thought, "This guy has played in a Grey Cup! He's a pro football player."

One of the nurses had John Doe's name from the police. "He's Terry Evanshen," she told the paramedics. Jim Jack was startled. Evanshen had been a boyhood hero of his. Jack had a distinct memory of watching a televised playoff game in Regina on a bitterly cold afternoon when Evanshen broke his leg. In Jack's mind's eye he could still see it, the men on the bench huddled in huge parkas, the plumes of condensation coming from their mouths when they spoke, the players crowded around the man on the ground.

"When you do the X-rays," he told the emergency staff, "you'll find he once had a fractured leg."

As nurses, a respiratory therapist, and a doctor swarmed around Terry, the paramedics left OR4 and settled down to write up the paperwork. When they finished, Jim Jack and Craig Jones replaced the equipment they had left behind with Terry and set out on their next call. Jack grinned at Jones. "Hey," he said. "We saved his ass. We just saved Terry Evanshen's ass."

TWO

Terry Evanshen returned from his three-week selling trip in Europe late on Saturday, July 2, 1988. When the airline limousine left him at his door, he carried his bags into the house, dropped them on the kitchen floor, and let out a comic's exaggerated sigh of relief. Lorraine, his wife, had waited up and wanted to hear about the trip, but he put her off, as she knew he would, and went straight upstairs. There, he unpacked his clothes, put them neatly away, and changed into comfortable pants and shirt. Terry is a very particular man. Then he returned to the kitchen for a cup of tea.

Lorraine remembers that he was in a wonderful mood, jubilant that the selling trip had exceeded his expectations. He had sold millions of dollars' worth of the attractive room heaters manufactured by Micromar International, his employers. He figured he qualified for almost two hundred thousand dollars in commissions. Pretty good for an ex-football player, and one of twelve

children raised in grim poverty in Montreal's toughest neighbourhood, Pointe St-Charles.

The next day Terry lounged around his new pool, getting
over jet lag and enjoying the chatter of his daughters, Tracy, eighteen, Tara, thirteen, Jennifer, eleven, and a twenty-year-old house-
guest, their cousin Charlie Dozois from Montreal, the son of
Lorraine's sister Clare. Tracy's new boyfriend, Joe Clark, nineteen,
had come from Toronto to spend the afternoon, and Terry paid
him warm attention. He entirely approved of this relationship.
Like a proprietorial Victorian father, he had formally given Joe his
blessing that he was welcome to see Tracy any time.

The news that day was full of the tragedy of an Iranian airliner
accidentally shot down by the United States Navy, and the
Church of England's anguish over the ordination of women. And
the heat wave was expected to break soon.

Monday morning Terry left for his office at Micromar International in Orono, a small town east of the farm, to tell the owners
the good news of the European orders. Once during the day he
phoned Lorraine, bursting to report how pleased his employers
were with him. He added that he expected to be home around
five-thirty.

The next time the family heard from Terry Evanshen was
the phone call taken by Jennifer, his youngest daughter, at about
a quarter to six. Terry was on his car phone to say he was on
his way, just approaching Brooklin, a small town only a few
kilometres from the farm. Did Lorraine want him to pick up
anything for dinner? Lorraine said no, and Jennifer conveyed the
message. Before hanging up, the little girl added from habit,
"Love you, Dad."

Lorraine checked the wooden picnic table on the awning-covered flagstone patio. She was proud of the way it looked, the perfectly matched placemats and napkins fresh and folded. The centrepiece was a bouquet of wildflowers Jen had gathered in a nearby field. Lorraine is fussy about appearances, her own and her household's. A pretty woman almost exactly the age of her husband, she is "four foot ten *and a half*" and beginning to round out. Her fine straight hair is cut in a blonde cap that lies close to her head and her hazel eyes are humorous under heavy dark brows. She's a devoted, impeccable housekeeper, and a fine and hospitable cook with a flair for desserts. Both Evanshens remember the poverty of their childhoods and rejoice in a well-maintained establishment.

Fifteen minutes passed with no sign of the Jeep. Lorraine's first thought about the puzzling delay was that Terry had stopped in Brooklin to buy a treat for dinner. Then, as more time went by, she decided he must have fallen into a conversation in a Brooklin shop and couldn't extricate himself. Then she wondered if he had also stopped for gas. Then, another ten minutes later, she made a worried call to his car phone. It rang but no one answered. Tara and Jennifer, growing restless, got her permission to saddle their ponies and go for a ride around the property. Joe, Tracy's boyfriend, needed a ride to the GO bus stop in Whitby so he could return to his night job in Toronto, but Terry still wasn't home with the Jeep. Unwilling to wait any longer, he and Tracy took the family's ancient truck with a horse trailer still attached, which Tracy found a hilarious conveyance.

Tracy was delayed on her return because the truck briefly broke down, but when she finally reached home her father still had not arrived. "This is kind of bizarre," she thought.

At seven Lorraine developed a terrible dread. She called the Micromar office. Doug Ridley, one of the two owners, was there. "Did Terry forget something and go back to the office?" she asked. He said no. When she told him about the mysterious delay, he was also concerned. It was completely out of character for Terry Evanshen not to be in touch with Lorraine to explain the holdup. "If you don't hear anything in another fifteen, twenty minutes, call me back," he said.

She called twenty minutes later. "Something is drastically wrong," she said. Doug Ridley agreed. He offered to drive the route Terry always took from office to farm and see what he could find.

It was well after eight-thirty when a police car turned in the Evanshen driveway and stopped beside the patio. Lorraine bolted upstairs crying, unready to hear what the visitors had to say. Tracy, a replica of her feisty mother, answered the door and assumed a belligerent stance that sprang from her own fears.

"Is this 6200 Coronation Road?" asked a uniformed policeman.

"Can't you read the mailbox?" Tracy responded curtly.

"Is this the Evanshen residence?"

"Yes, that's on the mailbox too." *Get to it!* She was thinking.

Ignoring her rudeness, the policeman went on, "Do you know a Terry Evanshen?"

Tracy could not control her irritation. "Yes," she said shortly.

"What is his relationship to you?" the policeman continued, unruffled.

"That's my dad. Now, what is going on here?"

"Where is your mother?"

"She's upstairs freaking out," Tracy shot back. "Will you please tell me what's going on?"

The policeman repeated. "Please get your mother. I need to take her to the hospital."

Lorraine had composed herself and was already back downstairs. When he saw her, the policeman said, "I'd like you to come with me to the hospital. Your husband's been in a very bad motor-vehicle accident."

Lorraine began to shake. It was hastily decided that her nephew Charlie should go with her for support, while Tracy would remain at home to look after her young sisters. Lorraine instructed Tracy to call Doug Ridley at the office, and their neighbours, Inez and Bob Piehl. As soon as her mother was out the door, Tracy went back into the kitchen, picked up some dishes, and threw them at the wall. Later, alone in the barn, she sobbed on the shoulder of her horse.

As the police car left the driveway, Lorraine saw Tara and Jennifer on horseback on a hill, silhouetted against the lavender evening sky and waving cheerfully. They thought Charlie had got himself into some scrape with the law, and both were amused. At the sight of her daughters, so innocently unaware that tragedy had struck, Lorraine burst into tears.

"How badly hurt is he?" she asked the policeman.

He answered, "I really can't tell you that." Lorraine concluded that Terry was dying, and clenched her jaw to avoid screaming.

A little after nine, the police car stopped in front of the sliding glass doors of the Oshawa General Hospital emergency entrance. One of the officers escorted Lorraine and Charlie into a tiny room to the right of the entrance, a spaced reserved for shocked relatives to receive bad news in private. Chuck Nash, who was waiting there, got to his feet. He had just informed Daryl Pertan, driver of the blue Chevy van, that he was charged with failing to stop at a red light. "There was no evidence to support any other charge than that," he later explained. "The charge would have been the same even if Mr. Evanshen had died." Pertan later was fined fifty-seven dollars and change for the offence.

Out of consideration, if circumstances permit, police officers who were at the scene of an accident involving a serious injury will make themselves available to the family to answer questions, so Nash had remained at the hospital after serving the warrant on Pertan. He was dreading what lay ahead. From the attitude of the paramedic, he expected that Terry Evanshen would not live. Nothing in police college manuals or his young life experience had prepared Nash for dealing with the raw grief of a newly bereaved family. He composed himself to say something neutral about his regret and sympathy, but when he saw Lorraine's stricken face, what came out was, "Ma'am, please accept my condolences."

Lorraine, rattled, snapped at him. "What are you talking about?" she demanded. "There's no way that he's dead." Nash, distressed, withdrew in confusion and left Lorraine in the hands of a nurse, who explained that Terry was being prepared for the operating room. "His injuries are very grievous and he's in pretty bad shape," the nurse said. "He will need a number of operations, but I don't know much more than that. You'll have to wait until one of the doctors is free to talk to you."

Lorraine felt her stomach wrench and came close to throwing up. When the nausea passed, she said firmly, "Where is the chapel?"

The nurse showed her to the hospital's spartan, non-denominational chapel, and Lorraine, a Roman Catholic, began to pray. She can grin about it now. "I did some tall talking to God," she says. "For an hour, or more. You lose track of time."

"Terry was lucky, in a way, and he wasn't," says Marian Timmermans, an emergency room nurse who was on duty in the trauma room where Terry was taken by the paramedics. She's a big woman with cropped, minimum-upkeep hair and a sardonic sense of humour. She is very sure of herself and competent to her bones. Emergency room nurses tend to think of themselves as an elite within the profession, and not without reason. The lucky part she was referring to was that paramedics were nearby when the accident happened and the hospital was so close.

The unlucky part was on that lovely July evening Terry lost his past and his civilized, affectionate self.

Hospital records show that Terry was unconscious throughout his four hours in the emergency room. No obvious reason for the coma could be seen, but clearly something unpleasant had happened to his brain. In any case, the probable brain injury was not the first concern of the emergency room team that night. Their attention was on Terry's left chest, which had been smashed to pieces. He had had a great fall, and they were supposed to put Humpty Dumpty together again.

Linda Moyle, the respiratory therapist on duty, relieved Jim Jack, who had continued to bag Terry all the way down the corridor and into the surgical trauma room. Moyle removed the mask and assisted the doctor, Erik Paidra, as he threaded an endotracheal breathing tube into Terry's mouth and down his airway, a process called intubation. Because the emergency room had no mechanical ventilator, she attached the tube to a bulb connected to an oxygen tank, settled herself on a stool, and commenced squeezing it rhythmically.

Marian Timmermans meanwhile cut Terry's clothes away and noted with professional interest that he was a well-muscled man who seemed in his early twenties. Youth and fitness were on his side, she thought. She inserted a catheter as Paidra pulled off the strips securing the sandbag, lifted it off, and looked at Terry's flailed and fluttering ribs.

Timmermans says of Paidra's skill as an emergency room doctor, "On a scale of one to ten, Paidra rates a nine-point-nine. And a ten from the Canadian judge. He's very, very good." Paidra, thirty-three, had finished his medical education seven years earlier. He is the son of two doctors, and his only sibling, a sister, also is a doctor. An affable, calm man with a stocky build and silky hair that falls to one side of his forehead, he has made emergency room duty his profession. The pressure and variety suit him, and his decision-making process is so quick the nurses have admiringly nicknamed him "Flash."

The emergency room team was moving into what they call "the ABCs" of emergency care: Airway, Breathing, Circulation. Paidra decided that Terry had a pneumothorax – a collapsed lung – but there was no time to confirm it with an X-ray. Much of the air that Terry was breathing in because of the bagging was leaking into the pleural sac that surrounds the lung. The first thing to do was to release that trapped air, drain off puddled blood, and give the crumpled lung space to expand. The doctor put a knife into Terry's left hemithorax between the ribs, pushed them apart, and poked his gloved finger into the opening he had created. He was feeling for the edge of the lung. Satisfied when he touched it, he withdrew his finger and sprayed in a bit of anaesthetic to dampen reflex reaction. Then he fed a tube down the hole and into the pleural cavity. He connected the other end of tube to a positive pressure machine so that air leaking from outside the lung could be sucked out.

He then sutured the tube to skin to keep it in place, ignoring the blood that poured from the rough wound. Incidental bleeding was well down the scale of worries at that moment. Under the rules of the ABCs, emergency room personnel have been known to ignore a leg that was facing backwards while they focussed on helping the person to keep breathing.

Paidra stepped out of the room and phoned the surgeon on call, Dr. Donald Sproull. A Scot in his early sixties trained in Glasgow, Sproull was a respected, experienced general surgeon noted for his air of skepticism and his unflappably sound judgement.

Timmermans glanced at Terry's right arm and saw that it was hugely swollen. She removed the needle Jim Jack had inserted while an IV nurse put two intravenous needles into veins in the left arm, one of them for saline solution and the other whole blood, the universal type O used when there isn't time to do a blood match. Because Terry's blood pressure was low, suggesting the onset of shock, the IV nurse used Pall tubing, which delivers great volumes of fluid.

Vital signs were being taken every ten minutes. To test Terry's reactiveness, Timmermans at intervals took his hand and spoke loudly near his ear. "Hello Terry," she would call. "You're in emergency. You've had an accident. Squeeze my fingers." Nothing. After a while she stopped trying to communicate. Nurses and the doctor kept checking Terry's hands. A wrist twisted a certain way not only indicates brain injury but the general location of that injury.

Each person dealing with Terry called out what was being done, and Angie Bosy, a serene, dark-haired nurse, had the harrowing, high-speed task of keeping track of times and procedures. Bosy was what emergency teams call "the charter." Accuracy is essential, since a medical chart is a legal document and the information on it vital to attending physicians, but the conditions for recording ER information are hectic. Timmermans's designated role was "the doer," the nurse who works on the patient, a task she relishes.

A portable machine was wheeled in to take X-rays of Terry's chest and spine. Everyone stepped back to give the radiologist room, but the risk of scatter radiation from portable units is considered negligible, and few left the room. Concern for the spine goes right along with the A in the ABC mantra. Marian Timmermans says laconically, "What's the point of doing all these great things to save the guy, and then you've made him a paraplegic?" Until the emergency team is assured that the top seven vertebrae are intact, they limit what they do. She and another nurse pulled Terry's arms down in line with his body in order to elongate his neck for the X-ray. Within five minutes the radiologist was back with the report that the spine showed no obvious damage.

The chest X-ray was quite another matter. It revealed that at least five of Terry's left ribs were shattered in several places, the diaphragm appeared to be ruptured, and the stomach was displaced into the chest. Maybe other organs were in the chest as well, crowding the left lung.

A technician came from the lab to draw blood. The space was becoming crowded. "A controlled tizzy," Timmermans called it. She finds the scenes of bedlam on the popular television series *ER* hugely amusing. Real emergency room ORs are almost quiet, and filled with concentration.

The radiologist took another X-ray of Terry's spine as insurance, and reported again that it seemed all right. Erik Paidra didn't like the grotesquely bloated right arm, which looked to him as if it was a developing compartment syndrome. Some of Terry's arm muscles, assaulted by the saline solution from the misplaced IV, were beginning to be strangled within their confining sheath of fascia. In time, the squeezing could choke the life out of them. Paidra judged that the fascia would have to be sliced open to relieve the pressure, but that wasn't his call.

At 6:37, there was good news. Terry was moving all four limbs in what Angie Bosy recorded as "spontaneous and purposeful movement." Clearly, the patient would not be paralyzed. Because Terry was beginning to thrash around with abrupt movements, he was given Valium, a tranquilizer. The sandbags supporting his neck were left in place as a precaution.

At 6:50, Timmermans had a question of the doctor. "Has he had his tetanus?" she asked. Paidra didn't look up. "Just give him one," he said tersely. Right, Timmermans thought, annoyed at herself. *Who is there to ask?* By then Terry was connected to machines to monitor his vital signs, which had stabilized. Angie Bosy noted in the hospital record that the bag on the catheter was showing blood in the urine. Paidra had done a rectal examination prior to inserting the catheter, to make sure that the bladder was intact, but maybe there was kidney damage. To check out that possibility he ordered a pelvic X-ray.

An operating room was being prepared for Terry by nurses and technicians who would consult with surgeons and the anaesthetist, Dr. Jane Brasher, to see what would be required. Don

Sproull, the general surgeon on call, arrived to take charge. Paidra, relieved of responsibility, left to deal with the backlog in the emergency waiting room, where impatient, frightened people were expressing their indignation at the slow service. Sproull, studying the patient, the X-rays and voluminous reports, decided he would need the help of a skilled thoracic surgeon. He placed a call for Dr. Maurice Pockey.

Pockey (pronounced *Po-kay*), a South African who now has his practice in Las Vegas, was the one doctors and nurses at Oshawa General would want for themselves if they needed a chest operation. They have seen him perform wonders on people with lung cancer, for instance, and he is known for his ferocious dedication to the well-being of his patients. As a colleague, however, his tone was that of an icy martinet. Timmermans, who got along fine with Pockey by barking back, was glad that the hospital's top man was coming to deal with this desperately injured patient.

As Sproull waited for Pockey, he had time to turn his attention to Terry's inexplicable coma. He checked the pupils of Terry's eyes for the telltale blown pupil but he saw they were still of equal size, though small. He had a hunch that there was blood behind the left tympanic membrane, possibly from a base-of-skull fracture. He could not be sure without a CT scan (computerized tomography), which was multi-angled technology only available elsewhere in the hospital. Sproull alerted Dr. Doug Waller, neurologist, that he would be needed.

At 7:30 a pelvic X-ray was done, and the radiologist reported that everything looked normal. At 7:55 Terry was obeying commands — *move your right hand, move your left leg* — but did not open his eyes. The operating room was still being prepared for eventualities known and unknown, but because the patient's condition had been safely stabilized, the delay caused no anxiety. Maurice Pockey arrived at 9:50, surveyed the supine man, and sniffed, "What a mess."

He took another look at the well-muscled patient. "This man's an athlete," he said approvingly. "Football," someone told him.

Pockey conferred with Sproull. Much of what had happened to Terry Evanshen's chest could be seen on the X-rays, but the surgeons had no information about the injured man's brain. They had to make a decision about priorities – should he be sent for the CT scan before the chest surgery? If the patient needed neurosurgery he would have to be transferred to a Toronto hospital, since Oshawa General did not have a neurosurgeon. Sproull and Pockey concluded that the chest surgery should have priority because of the risk of transporting an untreated person with such severe injuries. Immediately after the chest repair Terry would be sent for a CT scan of his head. If there was a fracture or a hemorrhage inside the skull, it would be Waller who would order Terry's transfer by fast ambulance to a Toronto hospital with a neurosurgery team.

Terry's left ankle and foot were swollen, so an X-ray was taken. It revealed the old football fracture that Jim Jack, the paramedic, had predicted, secured with a metal screw. Angie Bosy found a lull in the activity that allowed her time to list the valuables taken from the patient: a watch on a black band, a wedding ring, and his Grey Cup ring, which she innocently described as a "school ring."

The lab report came back, confirming that Terry's left diaphragm, the sheath of muscle which is the primary support of breathing, was ruptured. This tear had given room for his stomach and spleen to move up into his chest. Terry was wheeled to the operating room at 10:15, where the anaesthetist, Jane Brasher, prepared the unconscious patient much as she would have a conscious one, connecting him to a ventilator and deepening his coma so he no longer thrashed around. Thereafter, she closely monitored his vital signs, especially the indicators of brain activity.

Don Sproull then did a laparotomy, a long incision from bottom end of the sternum to the lower body, which opens the abdomen like gutting a fish. A drastic wound, it is done when surgeons don't know exactly what they will find and need plenty of room to look around. The incision revealed pools of blood in the abdominal and chest cavity, leaks from ruptured organs, and Sproull found that Terry's stomach, spleen, and some intestine had been violently dislodged and were nestled high in the chest, next to the heart and left lung. The spleen had three large tears. Since spleens are spongy matter that cannot be stitched, the organ had to be removed. Sproull did the splenectomy and repaired some damaged blood vessels in the stomach, daintily patting the stomach and other viscera back where they belonged.

Maurice Pockey then moved in to repair the damaged left lung, which now had room to inflate. When he was finished, he placed two drainage tubes through the left chest wall and then sewed up the diaphragm and arranged the broken rib pieces within mending distance of each another. Ribs, because they are encased in a sheath, will do that on their own: broken ends reach out for one another and make a tiny knob where they join. As a final flourish, Pockey removed some of the glass from Terry's left arm and face, and exquisitely stitched the wounds; a needle artist.

The surgeons had noted that Terry's right arm was continuing to swell and a pulsimeter could detect no pulse in the whitened fingertips of Terry's right hand. It meant that Terry's blood vessels were being crushed. If circulation could not be restored the arm might have to be amputated. Sproull had ordered someone to call the orthopaedic surgeon on call, Dr. Alexander "Sandy" Clark, a small, wiry Scot. Clark arrived while the abdominal and chest surgery was still in progress, and scrubbed hurriedly. Then he took a position out of the way of the other surgeons and made a long incision on the inner side of Terry's right arm from elbow to wrist. Cautiously, he deepened the incision until he found the taut fascia that was choking several muscle groups, and sliced it open. The relieved muscles burst through. Clark then inspected and palpated the arteries to get the blood moving again, and tacked back the edges of skin along the wound, covering the long gap of bulging muscle with a temporary dressing. The next day a plastic surgeon would cover the exposed flesh with a skin graft. As proof that the surgery had worked, the pulsimeter then found a pulse, though a weak one, in Terry's fingertips.

What else? The blood in the urine. Sproull had found no obvious damage to Terry's kidneys during his abdominal exploration. The educated guess of the surgeons was that his left kidney had been bruised in the collision, and this accounted for the bleeding. Sproull checked the urine bag attached to Terry's catheter and was reassured to see that it was showing decidedly less blood.

It was almost midnight. Apparently, they were done.

A CT scan of Terry's head was taken immediately after the surgery. Somewhat surprising to all, in view of the patient's deep coma, it showed no sign of a major intracranial bleed or skull fracture. Neurologist Doug Waller ruled that it was safe to keep Terry in the Oshawa hospital. The unconscious man was taken to the recovery room, where a watchful nurse was posted at his bedside. If Terry's condition remained stable over the next few hours, he could be moved to the Intensive Care Unit.

An Oshawa General respiratory therapist, David McKay, later reflected on the quality of Terry Evanshen's care that night. "You know," he said, "he was covered in horseshoes. At every step of the way, from paramedics to emergency to operating room, he got the best."

Lorraine remained in the chapel until after ten that night, knowing the nurse would find her when there was news. Charlie, her nephew, had phoned the girls to tell them their father was still in the operating room. When Lorraine emerged from the chapel and returned to the tiny private waiting room in emergency, a nurse joined her at once. "Is he going to be all right?" Lorraine asked. The nurse was candid. "We really don't know. We'll have a better idea in twenty-four hours." The partners from Terry's company, Doug Ridley and Ross Peat, came to see what was happening and insisted on staying with Lorraine. She was numbly grateful, though she was too distracted for anything more than desultory conversation.

Some time after midnight, Don Sproull, still wearing surgical greens, came into the room and sat down wearily. Lorraine was dazed as he recited everything that had been done, using terms that meant little to her. She waited politely until he was finished before asking what was uppermost in her mind, "Can I see him?"

He said no. Lorraine and Charlie and the others could move to a more comfortable room close to the Intensive Care Unit, where Terry would be taken soon, but it was better for her to wait to see him until that happened. "The next few hours are crucial," Sproull told her. "Just stay nearby."

Between three and four A.M. on July 5, Terry was moved to the ICU and a nurse came to fetch Lorraine. When Lorraine saw her husband, she was aghast. "His body had tubes and wires all over the place. His right arm was bandaged and looked like it had blown up. His head seemed swollen to me, there were bandages all down the front of him," she recalled, "and he was breathing with a ventilator." She leaned over to kiss his forehead and saw, to her horror, that the skin of his back looked navy blue. The colour must have been a trick of light: the stain was the runoff of the brown skin-sterilizing solution painted on Terry before the incision was made.

Lorraine sensed from the nurse's body language that she was in the way, so she stayed only a few minutes. Unless she thinks someone is trying to push her around, Lorraine is an obliging person, so it was natural for her to be accommodating. Besides, she had already reasoned that she might gain better access to Terry if the hospital staff saw her as someone who would not be trouble. Doug Ridley and Ross Peat, Terry's bosses, left soon afterwards, taking with them the exhausted Charlie.

During the rest of the night and into dawn, a nurse came for Lorraine every hour and led her to the curtained cubicle where Terry lay amid apparatus that looked more suited to a lunar landing than one man's life support. For the five minutes the nurses allowed, Lorraine sat in the only chair, holding Terry's hand and willing him to live. Her antennae sharpened by fear and fatigue, she suspected that the ICU nurses had low expectations of Terry's survival, but she had no such doubts. "He's loved, he's needed too much," she told the Fates. "He can't die." She silently lectured the still figure, "*Don't you dare die!* I'm not ready to let you go."

Morning came, and she phoned Tracy, making her voice sound confident and reassuring. At the end of her report, as a concession to reality, she admitted wearily to her daughter, "He's in really bad shape." Lorraine promised she would go home in a few more hours, give them all a hug, and grab a shower and a nap before returning to the hospital. Tracy said everyone at home was fine. She had told Terry's brother Gordon and Gordon's wife, Christine, about the accident, and they were coming to the farmhouse to help.

By mid-morning on July 5, several people had arrived, their faces full of concern. Bob and Inez Piehl, the Evanshens' neighbours, promised they would look out for the girls, and Gordon and Christine offered whatever other help Lorraine needed. One practical consideration was transportation. Lorraine didn't drive, so she would need rides between the farmhouse and the hospital. She was persuaded to go home on the spot. Once there, she hugged her daughters, struggling not to cry in front of them, and made a phone call to Vancouver, where Terry's mother, Aline, was staying with her daughter Patricia and Patricia's husband, Joe Russo. Patricia said she would be on the next plane to help look after the household, and Aline promised to follow.

News of the horrendous accident to the famous football player Terry Evanshen was all over the media that day, and the Evanshens' phone rang steadily with inquiries. Because it distressed her mother so much to repeat the ominous details, Tracy took over telephone duty. She sturdily and courteously informed anxious relatives and friends that her father was badly hurt, he was still unconscious, he could not have visitors, but he was holding his own. All the Evanshens firmly believe that doubt about oneself or any other Evanshen invites the devil to sup. Lorraine gave Tracy money for whatever supplies the household would need in the next few days, and apologized for the burden the eighteen-year-old was being asked to bear.

"It's a terrible responsibility I'm putting on you," she told her daughter, "but my place now is with Dad."

Lorraine showered and lay down, but found she couldn't sleep. She dressed and returned to the hospital, where Terry's dire condition was unchanged. Telephone calls followed her there, including one from the then prime minister, Brian Mulroney, a famously solicitous man. An excited nurse relayed the message to Lorraine, who was sitting at Terry's bedside. Lorraine knows Brian Mulroney from his days as trustee of the Schenley Awards for each season's most outstanding Canadian player in the CFL, a football honour that Terry won twice. She likes Mulroney, whom she calls Brian, and appreciated the call, but she said, "Tell him I'm with Terry right now and I can't talk to him."

That morning Terry was returned to the operating room, where Maurice Pockey performed a tracheostomy, a relatively simple operation which involves cutting a small hole below the vocal chords and into the trachea, after which a breathing tube is inserted, connected by clear plastic hosing to a ventilator. The intubation done the night before in the emergency OR was intended as a temporary measure, since that method of providing air irritates airways and makes it more difficult to feed the patient. David McKay, twenty-four, the lanky and self-possessed respiratory therapist called in that day, later explained that Terry's medical team thought it would be a long time before he would be able to breathe on his own. If ever.

At the same time as the tracheostomy was done, Dr. Elizabeth Simmons grafted skin over the wide swath of raw meat in Terry's right forearm, scraping a fine layer of skin, mesh-cut to make it stretch, from Terry's left thigh. A bronchoscopy was done on the left lung and some more puddled blood was removed. New X-rays now showed that Terry also had three broken ribs on his right side, but nothing needed to be done except wait for them to heal themselves.

Another CT scan of Terry's head showed small dark shadows in the frontal lobes where his brain had bounced against the skull during the accident. Since this seemed insufficient to explain the coma, Sproull and Waller speculated that Terry might have also have suffered hypoxia, oxygen deprivation – a good guess. Communication between doctors and paramedics must have been imperfect: Jim Jack could have informed them that Terry had been "blue as jeans" and ended their speculation.

So why was Evanshen still unconscious? Doug Waller, the neurologist whose responsibility this was, refused to get excited. He had checked with a prominent neurosurgeon in Toronto who confirmed Waller's own view that nothing could be done for Terry in another hospital that Oshawa General was not already providing, since neurosurgery was not indicated. Over the next thirty-six hours, Waller ordered a series of CT scans in order to catch the first ominous signs of bleeding or swelling, which would necessitate immediate intervention. However, nothing threatening seemed to be happening. While mild disruption appeared in the right thalamus and the frontotemporal lobes, these were slowly but steadily improving. Terry's brain apparently had been only lightly injured. Waller also ordered electroencephalographs (EEGs), measurements of the pattern of electrical activity in the brain. Terry's brain waves on both sides of his brain were what Waller described as "reasonably robust." All seemed well, considering the violence of the crash.

"When you have a high-impact head injury," Waller explains, "the skull stops but the brain is still travelling at the same velocity the person was moving. The brain just whacks into the skull. So in closed-head injuries you often get pulping and the brain swells. But Terry didn't show much of that. His brain looked almost completely normal."

Still, the man remained in a coma. Waller says, "He was basically a warm corpse, not even breathing on his own."

That passivity lasted only briefly. Though Terry continued to be unconscious, he soon became far from immobile. His increasing restlessness alarmed his nurses, particularly as he was an exceptionally strong man. Their fears were realized hours after the plastic surgery when Terry, apparently irate that something painful was happening to his right arm, ripped the bandages, the splint, and half the new skin graft clean off.

The plastic surgeon was notified at home, where she had just arrived by bicycle. "Not to worry," she told Lorraine cheerfully when she got back to the hospital. "I thought that might happen and I saved some extra skin." It was decided to postpone the second skin graft for a time, and the open wound was dressed instead. Terry wrists were tied to the sides of his bed with soft towels to prevent a recurrence. As further insurance, he was sedated. His violently agitated movements were threatening the healing of the long incision in his torso and the fat wound in his side where Erik Paidra had inserted his finger and then the life-saving tube.

Over the next few days, Terry's desperate efforts to escape his nightmares became an issue of great concern. Terry was suffering what has come to be labelled "ICU psychosis," a state of panic that seizes patients who, drifting just under consciousness and in agony, sense themselves to be in an incomprehensible and therefore dangerous place. Commonly, they try to escape despite the encumbering attachments to ventilators, heart monitors, and IVs, apparently indifferent to the pain they cause themselves. Nurses once found Terry, still in a coma, standing beside his bed, having somehow climbed over the raised sides. After that, his sedation was increased and Valium was added to the mix.

This solved one problem but created another. With Terry deeply medicated to keep him quiet, it became impossible to know how much the heavy drugs were contributing to his continuing coma. Efforts to lower the strength of the sedatives only resulted in Terry thrashing around again. A week after the accident, when sedation was slackened slightly, Terry got his loosely-bound hand free enough to pull out one of the two tubes Pockey had inserted to drain his chest. Another time he jerked out the feeding tube by which he was receiving liquid nourishment, and it had to be replaced in his right nostril. To prevent him removing his catheter, which he also kept trying to do, nurses kept him in underwear. Because Terry would pick at wires connected to monitors, or whatever else he could reach in the limited range afforded by the restraints, nurses tied a mitt on his left hand. His right hand was less mobile because of the splint on his arm to protect the open fasciotomy wound.

Nurses in every ICU shift made almost the same observation on the medical charts, "pt [patient] mumbling and restless." The next notation, not infrequently, was that sedation or tranquilizer was administered. A later entry, "pt sleeping peacefully," seemed drenched in some very anxious nurse's relief that the husky, agitated man at last was quiet.

Maurice Pockey was growing certain that the more serious assault on Terry's brain was oxygen deprivation, rather than the "pretty good whack," as he called it, that happened in the accident. Pockey observed astutely two days after the accident, "I think he'll wake up in another two to three days and will probably have minimal or no motor defects. But if he's had some hypoxia injury to his brain, it's much harder to say anything right now about his intellectual recovery." Some colleagues disagreed, and said so on the charts. The real culprit, they believed, was not hypoxia but the "blunt" blow that Terry's head had received. The truth was that no one really knew what had happened to Terry Evanshen's brain, not even Doug Waller, as skilled a neurologist as could be found.

When Lorraine took the girls into the ICU to see their father a few days after the accident, all three wept. "It was a real shock to them," Lorraine said. "They'd never seen their Dad when he wasn't bustling around, a real live wire." Jennifer, sobbing, said, "Daddy, I love you." Her father's stillness unnerved Tara, and she was further taken aback by the strangeness of her mother talking to the unconscious man as if she were conducting a normal conversation. Tracy was most distressed of all. She left the room crying, and threw up in the washroom. She was reluctant to see her father again until he was out of the ICU.

She was comforted by her boyfriend, Joe Clark, who at only nineteen was turning out to be a gem. After his night shift in the mail room at the *Toronto Star*, Joe regularly drove to the Evanshen farm, parked in the driveway, napped in the car until the household began to stir, and then drove Lorraine to the hospital. Tracy thought, "This is a good one. Better hang on to him. He's a keeper."

Over the next days, the younger sisters immersed themselves in horse shows, which proliferate in summer, both of them enjoying the competition for ribbons. By mid-July, with Terry still unconscious, all three girls were in Vancouver for a family reunion of the Evanshens that had been planned for months. Lorraine thought it best to keep them busy and distracted.

A doctor new to Lorraine turned up one afternoon at the bedside and said he feared Terry's right arm was "dead." Blood circulation had not returned to normal, he told her. "We might have to amputate. How much does he need that right arm?"

"Are you kidding?" said Lorraine sweetly. "How much do you need *your* right arm, doctor?"

Lorraine wept on the phone to one of Terry's closest friends, J.I. Albrecht, the one-time Montreal Alouette personnel recruiter who gave Terry the break that started his football career. Albrecht agreed with her decision to refuse permission for the amputation. "When Terry comes to he'll go through the roof if he doesn't have that arm," Albrecht told her.

Lorraine's eighteen-hour vigils continued, as day after day went by — and then a week, and then a second week. Seated by her husband, she could not help wondering what the future would hold for them both. Given Terry's pride and fierce independence, was survival at any price something he would really want? At her lowest moments she questioned herself. "If it turns out he's a vegetable, if it turns out he'll be in a wheelchair and helpless, I wonder if I have the strength to cope."

She had become the nurses' favourite visitor. "I know my place in a hospital," Lorraine says mildly. "I'm never pushy, never aggressive." As a result, the permitted five-minute visits every hour stretched into half-hour visits, and then into unlimited visits anytime. In appreciation of their care of Terry and consideration for her, Lorraine brought the ICU staff boxes of homemade cookies and cakes every day. Terry's brother, Gordon, equally grateful, once spent two hundred dollars on a basket of fruit for the nurses.

Aline Evanshen, Terry's spare, dark-eyed mother, alert and watchful as a bird, arrived from Vancouver and took over the domestic duties that Lorraine could no longer do. Occasionally she joined Lorraine in the long, deeply tiring vigils by the bed.

When Tracy, Tara, and Jennifer returned from Vancouver, they assumed responsibility for the barn chores, cleaning the stalls and feeding seven horses and ponies, three of them boarders. Their thoughtful contribution to their mother's peace of mind was that they never complained to her, though the work was relentless and exceedingly heavy, especially for the younger two.

On each visit to the hospital, Lorraine brought Terry the cards, letters, and telegrams that were pouring in from all over the country. "I don't know if you can hear me," she would say to the man in the bed, "but anyway I'm going to read you today's mail." Many cards came from football players who had been

Terry's teammates. Almost all spoke of Terry's renowned "fighting spirit," which was just what Lorraine was counting on to pull him through.

Sometimes she nodded off, her head on her arms against the railing at the side of his bed. Whenever she went home for a proper sleep, she didn't stay long. She didn't want to miss being there when he opened his eyes. Her daughters don't remember seeing much of her those weeks in July.

Lorraine still is emotional when she describes the care that Kathleen Lavis, one of the ICU nurses, took of Terry in that period. Lavis would wash him from head to toe, shave him to perfection, shampoo his hair and blow it dry, and care tenderly to the fast-healing cuts on his face and left arm from broken glass. Lorraine, deeply touched, said to her, "If he could, he would thank you for this. All his life it has meant a lot to him to be immaculate. How he looks is really, really important to him, and he would be so grateful for the care you are giving him."

What kept Lorraine going, her main comfort during the ordeal of Terry's hospitalization, was Doug Waller, the forty-eight-year-old neurologist. Cultured and well travelled, Waller is the son of Salvation Army missionaries and was raised in India. He is a good-looking burly man with a square-jawed, humorous face distinguished by warm brown eyes. His style is relaxed and friendly, that of a man at peace with himself, but he had some curious work habits. Marian Timmermans, the nurse in emergency, says that Waller "keeps vampire hours." She comments merrily, "Unless his ass is on fire, he's not going to get to the hospital before ten."

"I don't know when he sleeps," Timmermans adds, her eyebrows arched in incredulity. "He sees patients all day and makes his round at ten, eleven at night." He confesses ruefully that he is "a night person." He grins. "The explanation for the long hours I work probably borders on inefficiency."

He likes to say that he was "only a bit player" in the Terry Evanshen story. "My main contribution to his therapy was to prescribe some sleeping pills for Lorraine," he tells people. Lorraine smiles at this. His main contribution was his kindness, and besides, she never took the pills.

In 1976 Waller was the first full-time neurologist hired by Oshawa General. It is not hyperbole to say that he was the hospital's most beloved figure. Legends had grown around his displays of consideration. Nurses said he had never given any one of them a bad time, a quality that made him somewhat unique among his colleagues, and he was equally popular with patients and families because he gave the impression he never had anything more important to do than chat with them.

Every morning around one-thirty, Waller phoned Lorraine at the farmhouse. "I know you're there," he would begin. "The nurses say you just left the hospital." In a cosy, unhurried manner, he talked to Lorraine sometimes for as long as an hour, calming her fears and joking about the weight he was putting on because of the baked goods she was leaving in the ICU. When she asked what she could expect when Terry resumed consciousness, he said diplomatically that Terry would certainly be different. Probably he would be irritable and difficult for a while.

Waller doesn't believe it is helpful to leave families unprepared for the worst. He also told Lorraine frankly, "There's a big problem, all right. We have to be realistic. It's even possible that Terry might end up in a vegetative state, but I don't really think that will happen. We can't be hopeless at this stage. I don't want you to be without hope." His encouragement flowed more from his own sanguine nature than from the state of Terry Evanshen's real prospects. As Waller well knew, the longer Terry remained in a coma, the more likely it was that he would never wake up. Among themselves, doctors don't use such delicate language as "vegetative state." They say, "The man is a cabbage."

"Actually," Waller later admitted, "I started to get a little worried that he wasn't coming around."

"There's some damage to the frontal lobes," Waller explained to Lorraine, "and that area of the brain relates to concentration and memory, and behaviour. But we don't know how badly they are damaged because his brain is still a bit swollen. The brain takes a longer time to recover than any other part of the body. We'll just wait and see."

Despite the unprecedented pace in recent years of discoveries about brain function, the frontal area of the brain keeps many of its mysteries. Contrary information abounds. For instance, lobotomization, performed by sliding an instrument like an ice-pick between the eyeball and the eyelid and swiping it around inside the frontal lobes, was a routine treatment of mentally ill people for many decades until the mid-century. Indeed, the inventor of the brutal surgery was awarded a Nobel Prize. After the surgery a startling change of personality would occur: once-violent people became dazed and obedient zombies. On the other hand, virtuous clergymen who experience brain damage in that same area can become coarse and lewd. "Judgement is affected," Waller explained to Lorraine. "It can go either way."

Despite Waller's air of conviction, both he and Lorraine were under some pressure to move Terry to a teaching hospital in Toronto. His colleagues were growing more apprehensive the longer Terry remained unconscious, and her friends were telling her that Oshawa General was just a small-town hospital, shouldn't Terry be in Toronto where the real experts were? But Lorraine's faith in Waller never wavered. Waller, in turn, showed his confidence in Terry's recovery by calling in the Oshawa hospital's rehabilitation specialist, Dr. Mark Mason, to make a preliminary assessment. Mason was of the opinion that Terry's brain damage was more likely from the blow to the head than from lack of oxygen. But he added what had become the hospital's mantra: he couldn't be sure.

One early morning, Waller called Lorraine with good news. He had just been talking across Terry's bed to a nurse, and he asked her if she knew if Terry was right- or left-handed. Terry's right hand, still fettered loosely to the side of the bed, shot up. "You know what," Waller said to the nurse, "this son of a bitch can hear me."

Following that, one of the business partners brought an inspired gift, a cassette tape player and some of Terry's favourite country music. One day, with Ray Price on the tape deck, Lorraine was ecstatic to see Terry's toes moving, keeping time to the music. A few days after that she saw Terry mouthing the words of a song. The coma was lifting.

A few minutes at a time, and then for longer periods, Terry was being weaned from the respirator. At intervals David McKay and other respiratory therapists would warily disconnect the tubing, keeping a close watch on the blood-gas indicator as Terry managed a few breaths. When his breathing weakened they would reconnect the tubing. The next try, Terry would breathe on his own a bit longer than before, and so on, until he was breathing independently for long periods. On July 23, he was taken off the respirator.

Over that long process, McKay developed profound admiration for Lorraine. "We all had a lot of respect for her, and she was always appreciative and trusting with us. It was a very good relationship."

The drainage tube in Terry's chest was removed, and he began to open one eye, never both at once, and stare without comprehension at Lorraine and the nurses. One afternoon, somewhere at the beginning of the third week, Lorraine went home for a break. It was the first daytime one she had yet taken, but she was feeling desperately tired. The phone rang and when she answered it a man said, "Hi."

"Hi," she replied with little enthusiasm.

"Lorraine, it's Terry," said the man.

"Yeah, right," said Lorraine, annoyed at the prank.

"This is Terry," the man insisted.

Lorraine, now angry, said, "I don't know who you are, or what you think you're pulling, but I don't think this is funny." She thought she recognized the voice as that of Peter Dalla Riva, who played football with Terry in Montreal and had been calling almost daily.

"Peter," she said sternly, "I don't know if you're drinking or what's going on, but this is not a joke."

"I said it's Terry," the man said, raising his voice.

"Well, I don't believe you," Lorraine responded.

"Just a minute," the man said. A woman came on the phone and identified herself as a nurse Lorraine knew.

"It's true," she told Lorraine. "It is Terry."

"I'll be there in a minute," Lorraine yelled. *Damn him*, she thought, *he would wake up the only time I'm not there.*

She found Terry sitting in a wheelchair at the nurses' station. Lorraine bent down and hugged him. He didn't react. She pulled back in surprise and saw from his face that he hadn't the faintest idea who she was. He looked away in complete disinterest. He already had forgotten the phone call and the name that nurses had coached him to say.

They'd told him he had a wife. He had forgotten that too. In any case, *what's a wife?*

THREE

It was no surprise to the staff at Oshawa General Hospital that Terry Evanshen didn't recognize Lorraine. The man had been in a disastrous accident during which he sustained what they thought was a mild brain injury, and a degree of temporary amnesia was to be expected following such trauma. The usual pattern is that people in such mishaps will have a period of confusion and post-traumatic amnesia (PTA) for a few hours or days after regaining consciousness. Except for the blank spot of the incident itself, when the brain either can't retrieve the memory of the deeply shocking incident or else it was too overwhelmed at the time to record it at all, people usually resume their lives with only the memory of a headache to show for it.

Long-lasting amnesia is a comparatively rare phenomenon. Only ten percent of closed-head injuries involve some degree of memory loss, and almost all of these have some of both major categories of amnesia: anterograde amnesia, which is impaired ability to store new memories, and retrograde amnesia, the memory of one's past before the injury. People with anterograde amnesia compensate with lists to remind them what they have to do next, but in time most recover their ability to make plans and remember them. The brain, on its own, seems able to construct circuits to substitute for damaged ones, or it may even send a flood of new neurons to help with repair work. Retrograde amnesia, the loss of some or all of one's past, is less likely to reverse itself. Brains seem able to cope fairly well with the task of making alternative circuits and repairs so that new-memory mechanisms function again, but when prior memories vanish, brains seem unable to recover. The cells and connectors where old memories lie throughout the brain have simply been blasted out of existence. When the brain has been injured in the fibrous uncinate fasciculus, which connects the frontal and temporal lobes, the memories may still be intact but the brain can't find them.

James McCoubrey, then vice-president of the Canadian Broadcasting Corporation, suffered a car accident in 1998 which left him with his head buried in snow for so long that he experienced a degree of asphyxia. McCoubrey was a long time without any understanding of where or who he was, and when he recovered from that disorientation he found he had lost the memory of five years of his life. A bilingual Chicago Blackhawks hockey player, J.P. Dumont, knocked himself out during a National Hockey League game early in the season in 1999 and for a period afterwards was unable to speak English.

In almost all clinical experience, people with retrograde amnesia never lose everything. Recent past may be gone, but usually something remains of early life. One patient of Doug Waller, for instance, forgot her whole life after her marriage but she retained perfect recall of her childhood and youth. People with Alzheimer's disease may not know what they did that morning but they can recite an old recipe for tea biscuits, or the words to a hymn they sang in childhood. The British actor Stanley Holloway died at age ninety-one and just before his death observed sadly, "Things that I did fifty years ago I find I can remember, but things I did five weeks ago I have no idea."

Each year half a million people in North America have a closed-skull brain injury, the most common cause of significant neurological disorder, but most of them recover their ability to remember. However, the behaviour changes that can follow such injuries may not be happy ones, particularly if the frontal lobes suffered damage. While memory usually returns to working order, personalities may not. Typically, such brain-injured people are tactless, irritable, uninhibited, intolerant of frustration and noise, egocentric, impulsive, and have repetitive and fixed habits.

The expectation at the Oshawa General Hospital that summer was that Terry would be a grumpy man for a while but that this would dissipate in time. No one could imagine that he would lose, permanently, every bit of his personal history and also not be able to form new memories. The medical staff reasoned it simply wasn't possible to have that much brain damage and still live.

"How can so much memory be erased and he wasn't knocked off?" Doug Waller wonders. The neurologist was astonished by his patient. "Terry could have died, but he didn't. The reason he's alive is that people got him breathing again. And also credit is due to Terry. He just has a different light bulb than other people."

What the doctors did not realize for many months was that the minor damage to Terry's frontotemporal lobes that appeared on the CT scan was only the beginning of his problems. Specific areas of these lobes which gave him emotional depth had been damaged, but the real wreckage was undetectable by the technology available at the Oshawa General. Terry's brain had suffered two additional devastating blows. One was the lung and rib damage that resulted in protracted oxygen deprivation, which killed millions of neurons throughout his brain. "It's not like you have a healthy brain with a few holes in it," Waller commented later. "The asphyxiation Terry suffered extended everywhere in his brain and affected key circuits." The other bad news was the violent shaking his head had taken as he was hurled out the back window of his Jeep to land face-down fifteen feet away.

The brain is made up of neurons, which are cells with a "tree" on one side whose many branches are dendrites, two-way communication specialists, and a tail-like sprout called an axon which may have as many as ten thousand terminals, all of them message-senders. The twists and torque Terry's brain suffered in the split seconds of his trajectory destroyed and rearranged the white-matter circuitry that facilitated the memory and personality and value system Terry had spent forty-four years assembling.

The destruction of brain cells from hard shaking has a name: diffuse axonal injury (DAI). Axons all over the brain are stretched and then snap, which destroys their ability to send messages; since they have been rendered useless, they atrophy. "A small injury that puts you in a coma doesn't affect the parts of the brain that store information," Doug Waller explains. "They are sitting there intact, waiting for the switch to come on. People who get a little hemorrhage in the brain stem that knocks out their main switch will wake up and be fine, but people who have a diffuse axonal injury have something different. It doesn't matter if the switch goes on or not, all the storage is gone. Lack of oxygen, as well, would affect the whole brain."

In the 1980s, sophisticated technology for seeing such damage was either unknown, or beyond the financial resources of all but the country's largest teaching hospitals. Brain destruction from hypoxia or DAI had to be deduced rather than observed. One indicator of DAI, for instance, is the speed the person was travelling and how hard the stop was (a fall of more than six feet will cause plenty of problems). Another is whether unconsciousness was immediate without a prior lucid interval, which is not promising in terms of recovery. The third indicator is the Glasgow Coma Score, used to assess the severity of a coma. Less than a six, and a good recovery will happen only twenty-one per cent of the time. Terry's Glasgow Coma Score was three, the lowest before death. Terry, in fact, had all three defining elements of DAI at its worst.

According to Dr. Douglas I. Katz, a Boston neurologist, the rate of recovery from DAI depends on the severity of the damage. Progress toward normalcy is liable to stall at any phase, he warns, including an early one. A permanent vegetative state is entirely possible. Shaken babies, for instance, frequently become unconscious, and many die.

In Terry's situation, DAI was only one part of the assault on his brain. "When you put together a flailed chest and a brain injury, it isn't one plus one equals two," comments Dr. Ronald Kaplan, one of the Canada's most experienced neuropsychologists. "In Terry's case, one plus one equalled a hundred."

Kaplan is a solidly built, greying, calm man who, with his wife, operates a large brain-injury clinic in Hamilton. He explains that after Terry's brain took the small bang that caused it to rock inside his skull from front to back, and shook it like a martini, it would have immediately commenced repair work by ordering up an increased blood flow to access more oxygen. But because Terry's lung was not functioning properly, the extra blood his brain needed contained almost no oxygen, so it was useless.

"The brain injury he received might have been minor, and there could have been a complete recovery," Kaplan says, "but the oxygen the brain needed to start the repair wasn't there. Instead of a recovery, there was a catastrophe."

DAI does its greatest havoc in susceptible locations such as the frontal lobes, which make up one-third of brain mass. Lying behind the forehead and above the eyes, frontal lobes perform the brain's most polished skills. That part of the brain is now the focus of intense and fascinating study, and neuroscientists are beginning to appreciate the tremendous and critical role that frontal and temporal lobes play in personality, intelligence, memory storage, and memory retrieval.

Frontal lobes spurt in growth between birth and age seven, the period when the human brain almost doubles in size, and finish expanding in the late teens and early twenties. These lobes, neatly parted into two as though a comb had been passed over them, are intricately connected to all other parts of the brain. They contain or are responsible for the brain's most highly developed faculties of concentration, wisdom, deductive skills, aspiration, empathy, philosophical beliefs, sociability, imagination, and affection.

All these refinements are acquired by adults through a process of accretion and substitution that begins imprinting itself on behaviour from infancy. The inclination to be generous, for instance, is something toddlers acquire when their own needs are well met and affectionate caregivers urge them to share toys. Children raised this way or who become adults determined to turn themselves into considerate people will store an inclination to be kind either in their frontal lobes or accessed from elsewhere by its connectors. The frontal lobes, in a real sense, become custodians of personality and whatever kind of social conscience adults achieve. They are the seat of everyone's complex and highly individual identity. Accordingly, when frontal lobes are damaged, the consequence often is a decline in the civilities the person managed to acquire in a lifetime and a reduction in the ability to control temper, which is one of civility's best tricks.

Because the assaults on Terry's brain from DAI, oxygen deprivation, and possibly a reduced blood supply to the brain were not observable on the Oshawa General's CT scan, most of the professionals treating Terry waited confidently for normalcy to return. They knew his coma had been unusually long for such a mild frontal brain injury, but they thought that the heavy sedation he had received was partly responsible. In any case, the rule-of-thumb is that a two-week coma will be followed by about nine weeks of muddled thinking and then clarity is restored.

If they were wrong, and Terry's behaviour was somewhat strange, the worst of it might be the confusion his family and friends would experience because Terry would be an altered person although he looked exactly the same. Most people who had known him before would think that nothing much had happened to him, leaving them no explanation for his irritability and rudeness. In *The Working Brain*, a classic text by the Aleksandr Romanovich Luria, a Russian considered by many to be the twentieth century's greatest psychologist and a pioneer in brain function, the author observed sorrowfully that damage to the frontal lobes may not be noticeable to others during a casual encounter but it is a devastation, a "profound disturbance of the whole structure of human conscious activity." Dr. Catherine Mateer, a clinical neuropsychologist in Victoria, B.C., and a world authority on cognitive rehabilitation, observes that frontal lobe damage frequently leaves people with their intellect and language skills unimpaired. The result is that "frontal lobe deficits present a perplexing and frustrating paradox to professional and layperson alike."

One of the world's earliest and most arresting demonstrations of the role frontal and adjacent temporal lobes play in personality occurred in Vermont in 1848. Phineas Gage, a railway worker, was leaning over a stick of dynamite when it exploded, driving a tamping iron into his face below his left cheek, right through the medial frontal lobes of his brain and out the top of his head. He walked to the cart that took him to hospital and seemed perfectly fine, except for a dramatically altered disposition. Gage had been a friendly and quiet man, but after the spike went through his head he became quarrelsome and nasty. People shook their heads and said, "No longer Gage."

A healthy adult brain is a misshapen, glossy, wet, pink blob of jelly weighing about three pounds and creased with deep folds like a walnut. It is softer than raw liver. When pathologists in an autopsy pluck out a fresh brain, it sags between their fingers. The brain is packed with about a hundred billion neurons, and information moves between the neurons by means of neurotransmitters, electrochemicals which enable data to leap across the gaps, called synapses. The energy generated by this busy process is sufficient to make a twenty-watt bulb glow.

To perform its astonishing tasks, the brain needs a great deal of oxygen, much more than its share. Though it takes up less than three percent of body weight, the adult brain uses twenty percent of the body's oxygen intake, day and night. This makes it the organ most vulnerable to oxygen reduction, a weakness exacerbated by the brain's regrettable lack of an oxygen back-up system to help it through an emergency. When a brain is deprived of oxygen for only ten seconds, unconsciousness occurs.

Frontal lobes, especially the right one, associated with creativity, are busy parts of the brain, and therefore particularly demanding of a constant and rich flow of oxygenated blood. Because they are highly vulnerable to reduced blood flow, the frontal lobes are easily damaged if something interferes with the blood supply, such as an hypoxic-ischemic injury, a combination of low oxygen and reduced blood flow seen most commonly following drowning or cardiac arrest. Another area highly susceptible to lack of oxygen is the hippocampus in the medial temporal lobe deep in the brain, which is the chief intake centre for acquiring new memories. Magnetic resonance imaging (MRI) has been used to watch activity in the hippocampi, specifically the part called the entorhinal cortex, of people with Alzheimer's disease. They found not much going on.

Memory-damaged old people ask, "Where am I?" Someone explains and they nod as if comprehending. Then they ask, in exactly the same interested tone, "Where am I?" Their hippocampi simply could not record the answer.

The functions that the brain performs instinctively, as on automatic pilot – movement, appetite, rage, fear, and sensory perception – survive age, oxygen deprivation, and other disasters quite handily. The basal ganglia right above the brain stem, which developed early in human evolution and rule movement, are relatively resilient to trauma. This explains why Terry was able to walk and speak after he regained consciousness, though he did not know his own name. His balance was uncertain and his words were slurred and sometimes incomprehensible, both states not unlike the behaviour of a toddler, but the fundamental functions of speech and movement were still there.

What did not emerge for a long time after Terry left the hospital was that the complex and devastating damage his brain sustained had resulted in combined losses rarely seen: total and intractable retrograde amnesia which knocked him back to the emotional level of a raging two-year-old, and a severe degree of anterograde amnesia.

The last, as Terry was to discover, was the worse. As Dr. Richard Restak, American neurologist, observed about such massive memory loss in *The Brain*, "Although both types of memory disturbances can devastate a personality, the lack of ability to form new memories is by far the more disabling."

No clinician who has examined Terry Evanshen – and he has been seen by dozens – has ever encountered such severe memory damage, though such cases are not unknown. Dr. Sandra Black, who heads the division of neurology at Toronto's Sunnybrook Health Science Centre and is a leader in the field of cognitive neurology, once encountered a man with such a loss much like Terry's, but unlike Terry, he became a docile person. Dr. Donald Stuss, a pre-eminent neuropsychologist who heads Toronto's Rotman Research Institute at the Baycrest Centre for Geriatric

Care, has written about a man who lost all his previous memories after sustaining brain damage in a bicycle accident, but this person had almost normal ability to acquire new information. It turned out that his uncinate fasciculus was torn.

A factor in the drastic degree of Terry's deficits may have been his career as a professional athlete. Though controversy still rages about this, some researchers are convinced that contact sports such as boxing, hockey, soccer and, especially, football – with its hard tackles on frozen ground – cause mild but incremental brain damage even if the athlete is never knocked unconscious. Much of the work in the field of mild multiple head injuries is being done in California, where football teams provide a steady stream of research subjects, and such investigations have resulted in return-to-play guidelines now in place in the National Hockey League and National Football League to help determine when it is advisable for a head-injured athlete to stay on the bench, or retire from the sport.

Lorraine Evanshen says that before the accident her husband never exhibited any signs of mild brain damage, such as memory lapses or unaccountable bursts of rage when he was fatigued. Still, many neuropsychologists would consider Terry to be more vulnerable to serious brain impairment following trauma than a person of similar age and fitness who had never been tackled to the ground. As early as 1962, a report by C. Symonds in the respected British medical journal *Lancet* stated, "it is questionable whether the effects of concussion, however slight, are ever completely reversible."

For example, the speculation is that Mohammed Ali suffered Parkinson's disease earlier and more severely than he would have if his brain had not experienced so much battering in the ring. Previous head injuries also seem to be a factor in the onset of Alzheimer's disease, though they are not the main one.

Dr. Mark Lovell, a Detroit neuropsychologist who is consultant to the National Football League and the National Hockey League, gives a "conservative estimate" that every year in North America approximately one hundred thousand football players suffer brain injuries. Fourteen years of being hit by heavy men every time he caught the football may have set Terry Evanshen up for his sad fate.

It is difficult to pin the blame on any one of the factors that caused the mayhem in Terry Evanshen's brain, whether it was the blow to his frontal lobes, or the asphyxiation that might have been combined with a blood flow inadequate to wash out impurities, or the diffuse axonal injury, or whether football contributed at all to the disaster. The reality is that the combination had appalling consequences for a football hero who on a sweet summer evening was happily headed home to barbecue a steak.

He lost, permanently, the first forty-four years of his life, and with it, his ability to be a sensitive, reasonable person. Gone was the man who came from a poor, fists-up background and received only a modest education, but through diligence, quick wits, and charm had become the proud possessor of an impressive country estate. Gone was the warmly affectionate man devoted to his generous-hearted wife and three sparkling daughters. Gone as well was the keen, irresistible salesman with a bright future.

All those splendid Terry Evanshens perished in the sun-bleached weeds beside a smashed Jeep.

FOUR

Aline Evanshen, Terry's mother, now in her late seventies, knows a lot about the person Terry was as a child, although it is not always easy for her to remember particulars about any one of her offspring when she had twelve to raise, each of them born about two years apart. Sometimes they blur together in her mind.

The size of her brood owed little to Roman Catholic family planning practices and everything to the wilfulness of her husband, John Evanshen, who wished to sire as many children as he could, preferably all of them male. In the Evanshen household, his word was law. He kept his family in line with displays of roaring rage that cowed his tough, street-smart sons and daughters, and his French-Canadian wife as well.

John Evanshen ordered up his bride like a man purchasing a good pair of boots – not too hard on the eyes and built for wear. He spotted Aline Belisle, as she was then, when she was sixteen. Born on August 25, 1921, Aline was the third of seven children in a French-Canadian family made desperately poor by the Depression. The Belisles had moved from Abitibi, a pulp and paper town in Ontario's northland, when the mill closed and they were in Val-d'Or, a Quebec mining town, where they barely scraped by. Aline, who left school in grade three, was working as a domestic. John Evanshen, then nineteen, met her when he made a grocery delivery one day to the Belisle household and noticed Aline warming herself by the wood stove in the kitchen.

She spoke no English and he spoke no French, but that didn't deter him. He announced to Aline's father that he wanted to marry her, and that was that. She didn't even like him. He was a burly, abrasive man and not particularly good looking, with the big-boned face of his Slavic heritage and hard green eyes. Though he was not to her taste, she went along with the arrangement, hoping he would be her ticket out of poverty and toil.

It never did work out that way. Their first baby, Steven, was born nine months later, but poverty and toil were there from the beginning of the marriage. By the time Steven came along, Aline had learned enough about John Evanshen to understand his rough ways. His mother died when he was young and his father put him in an orphanage for a while, retrieving him when he married a mail-order bride sent from the Ukraine. Aline says of his step-mother, "She was a real witch. Mean to children. It made me feel sorry for him. I loved him more because he wasn't loved at home."

Evanshen, Aline says, is a shortened form of Evanshenishyn, the name Terry's Ukrainian grandfather bore when he came to Canada. Aline discovered that her new husband had no intention of learning French and, indeed, he declared that he detested everything French. Forbidden to speak her only language in his presence, she rapidly acquired English, though her speech retained a Gallic lilt.

The couple settled in Timmins briefly and then, following whatever jobs John could find, moved first to Toronto and finally to Montreal's Pointe St-Charles district, where rents were cheap. Pointe St-Charles, in southwest Montreal, represented urban poverty at its deepest. Populated by a mixture of English- and French-speaking blue-collar workers, the neighbourhood offered jobs for some in a glass factory and a railway repair yard – both since closed. The Point, as it is called by Montrealers, was renowned at that time for its brawling street gangs and the thieving ways of its belligerent young males. In recent years it has undergone a half-hearted effort at urban renewal, but Pointe St-Charles is still a dispirited, weedy community of sagging row houses, second-hand clothing stores, food banks, and abandoned factories with dirty windows.

This is where John Evanshen brought his teenaged wife and young sons. "He was some kind of a nut," Aline says of her husband, who died in 1982. She means he was a nomad, moving restlessly from job to job. Sometimes he was an inventor, and sometimes a gold prospector – he often described himself as a geologist – and sometimes a taxi driver. She never knew what he would do next. "A flim-flam man," Lorraine's sister calls him. To give the family stability of sorts, Aline for a while ran a shabby café on Wellington Street, a thoroughfare in Pointe St-Charles, where she cooked burgers and fries. The Evanshens, adding a new baby to their family every two years, lived in small, dark rooms in the back.

Aline loved being pregnant. Bearing children was never a hardship for her, but in twenty-four years, she had twelve babies: eight sons and four daughters. Somewhere in that celebration of fecundity she longed to call a halt. She consulted a doctor and asked about contraception. He told her to forget it. If she wanted to stop having babies, she should leave her husband.

Aline has to pause and think which child was Terry. "Let me see. Steven, Fred, Gordon, ah, and then Terry. He was the fourth." Terrance Anthony Evanshen was born on June 13, 1944, in a back room at the hamburger joint. Lorraine Evanshen, whose family lived nearby in poverty equally dire, believes that after Aline's babies were delivered by a doctor making a house call, Aline would get up immediately from the birth bed and go back to flipping hamburgs. Aline, who is sensitive to any suggestion that she lacks refinement, denies this indignantly. She says she rested a while after her babies were born and *then* went back to work.

Terry, as it turned out, was the next-to-smallest of John and Aline's eight handsome sons, but he was the most proud, ambitious, and almost absurdly particular about his appearance. Possessed of superb physical coordination, he threw himself into sports with a fanaticism that swept him to the forefront of whatever game he played. In keeping with his emerging status among his peers, he refused early in his boyhood to go to school with clothes that needed mending, and as a teen even balked at wearing jeans. Indeed, he checked each morning that the crease of his trousers was straight, and he ironed his clothes himself to make sure the job was done right. He seemed constitutionally unable to accept any flaw in his armour, and this included ever admitting he was in pain or ill. From early childhood, he kept to himself whatever discomfort he suffered. When he broke his leg at age seven or eight in a school accident, he wouldn't deign to use crutches.

Lorraine's parents, George and Susan Galarneau, knew the Evanshens slightly and regarded them somewhat askance as a tumultuous lot. Not that the Galarneaus' life was any easier. At his most prosperous, George Galarneau earned a modest income delivering groceries by horse and wagon for his father's grocery store, where the family lived upstairs. When the store failed in the Great Depression because people could not pay their food bills, he was lucky to find a low-pay job as a night watchman at the railway repair yard.

Like the Evanshens, the language of the Galarneaus and their eight children was English. Susie was Irish-Catholic, as were many of the anglophones of Pointe St-Charles, and George, who was comfortable in both French and English, deferred to her. Besides, he reasoned, English-speaking children had a better chance at employment, a grievous state of affairs that contributed greatly to the Point's teenage gang wars: French boys besetting *les maudits anglais* and being ambushed in turn by packs of English youths.

The birth of Lorraine, the youngest of the Galarneau children, came as a shock to her mother. Susie, at forty-five, felt comfortably finished with childbearing. Her youngest, Clare, was fifteen and the only one still at home. The others had died young or else were adults and out on their own. Feeling unwell one summer day in 1944, Susie consulted a doctor who told her in a minute flat that she was seven months pregnant. Since Susie was obese, she showed no sign of her advanced condition. Lorraine Paula Mary was born on August 11, 1944, two months after Terry Evanshen. Five months later George Galarneau died, leaving the family penniless.

Clare Galarneau, a short (four foot ten), industrious, generous-hearted woman who is strongly imbued with a sense of family and social responsibility, promptly left high school and went to work to support her mother and baby sister. "There really was just myself, Lorraine, and Mom," Clare says, adding fondly, "Lorraine was a beautiful and smart little thing." Clare, in truth, raised Lorraine. Susie was far too heavy to go walking with a toddler, so outings from the beginning were Clare's responsibility. The family lore is that one afternoon in nearby Margaret Bourgeoys Park, two babies – Lorraine and Terry – played together on a blanket.

When Clare married Charles Dozois in 1951, the couple continued to play a parental role in the life of the little girl. Charles, a kind man known to all as Chuck, is an avid amateur photographer and took pictures of the enchanting child as she grew. Lorraine and her mother lived in a walk-up flat on Charron Street where the walls were thin as tissue paper and the ceiling so flimsy that sometimes, when there was a party upstairs, plaster fell on their bed as they slept. They survived on a bit of money Susie made preparing meals for the priests in the rectory and what was called the "needy mothers' pension." Lorraine's sisters each contributed ten dollars or so a month to help with the rent.

Everyone else they knew was just as poor, so they were not humbled by their privations. And they had always had the solace of their religion: mother and daughter attended Mass regularly and took seriously all Roman Catholic observances. For sure, Friday was fish day: fried patties made of tinned salmon and left-over mashed potatoes.

The ethic of the household was to help others. Susie believed in giving, and Lorraine came to take it for granted that all people have a natural and unalterable obligation to assist one another.

When the time came, Lorraine went to St. Gabriel's Academy, an all-girls Roman Catholic school taught by the Sisters of the Holy Cross. She says, still awed by those vigilant and dedicated nuns, "They were something else. They could terrify you." Terry, meanwhile, was at the Pointe St-Charles all-boys Catholic school, Canon O'Meara, where he was taught by the Christian Brothers. The two children might have been aware of another, living so close, but the segregated schools and Terry's obsession with sports kept them apart until they were about twelve and beginning to hang out at the local community centre.

Pointe St-Charles, for all its shortcomings, had one wonderful asset that affluent neighbourhoods often lack, a Boys' and Girls' Club, a bustling, well-staffed recreation and crafts centre for young people. The centre drew impoverished adolescents from miles away to its after-school programs and weekend activities. Terry saw Lorraine there and apparently was dazzled by her, a tiny, assured, practical person with a bubbling sense of humour. He began to pursue her aggressively.

He took manly responsibility for walking her to and from the centre, a forty-minute hike through the hazardous French-speaking neighbourhood. On those occasions when he was busy with one of a multitude of his athletic activities, he conscripted friends for escort duty. Lorraine, an independent-minded person even as a child, was annoyed. She told him to leave her alone, but he kept on watching out for her.

Out of curiosity, she went one day to watch him play hockey and was smitten. "Tutti Evans," as he was known in the Point, was an extraordinary sight. Handsome, adept, and brave, he was the team's scoring champion. Lorraine's quickened interest encouraged Terry. He started hanging around her flat after school. "I think he was attracted to the tranquility," Lorraine comments. "Our place was always peaceful and quiet, while his place was chaos, children everywhere. They had moved to a small flat on St. Madeleine at the time. As I remember it, all the kids were in one bedroom, with a curtain between the boys and the girls." Her sister Clare comments, "I don't think that Evanshen family ever knew what it was like to sit down together for a meal."

"Stay away from her," Aline cautioned her son. "Have you seen her mother? *Fat!* Lorraine's going to look just like that." The Galarneaus were not much more enthusiastic about the Evanshens, who had a reputation in Pointe St-Charles for unruliness, and some of the boys were not unknown to the police. Clare cautioned her mother, "Don't let Terry come to the house so much."

Neither child paid any attention to the elders. Terry was stuck on Lorraine, and Lorraine, in turn, was flattered to be pursued by the popular, confident boy who sometimes, to please her, even accompanied her to Mass. As they grew older, they became regulars at the Friday night dances for younger teens at the Boys' and Girls' Club and then moved on to the Saturday night dances for the older ones, where CJAD radio disc jockey Mike Stevens was the emcee. They danced every dance together. That was Terry's idea, not Lorraine's. Watching her dance with someone else was not his notion of a good time.

Aline does not remember Terry's boyhood home as being in the least discordant. In her account of the Evanshen household, she summons up scenes of harmony and goodwill, with outings to the park or a beach, pots of wholesome vegetable soup on the stove, and everyone always spic and span. Policemen at the door are not part of her narrative, nor are the times when she was fed up with the lot of them and chased them out of the house with a broomstick. What undoubtedly was true about their circumstances was that Aline waged a heroic struggle to present a respectable front to the neighbours. Keeping her house spotless was only the beginning of her battle to defend the Evanshen reputation. Aline, a woman who can sense slights undetectable to others, still believes that the Point held her in contempt for having so many children. Her efforts to maintain her dignity could not have been easy, especially whenever the family had to move because of problems paying the rent, and John Evanshen was an argumentative, stormy man whose shouting could be heard over great distances.

One of the daughters, Judith Evanshen Perry, is a crisp, straightforward woman in her early forties who possesses the incandescent Evanshen smile. She now lives in Calgary with her husband, Bernard, and she says her father was firm with the boys but more indulgent with his four daughters. She remembers him packing his car with as many children as he could round up and taking them all to the park for the day. That's the way Tracy Evanshen remembers him too. When she was a small child living in Montreal, her grandfather was just about the kindest and most loving person she knew. She called him Pappy, and he often came to visit, taking up his post under the fruit trees in their back garden, where he would feed the squirrels and patiently peel apples for baby Jennifer to eat. The family remembers that John doted on shy, quiet Jennifer, and even volunteered to change her diaper. Aline was flabbergasted.

The Evanshen family history is full contradictions, depending on which Evanshen is doing the telling. For instance, Terry believes that he started to smoke a pack or two a day at age eight and gave it up three years later, after becoming violently ill following a sports jaunt to New York when he travelled all day in a closed car full of smokers. He no longer remembers this on his own, of course, but Lorraine heard him tell the story many times in their years together before his accident and has described it back to him. Aline Evanshen and Judith Evanshen Perry, the youngest of her four daughters, however, stoutly deny that it ever happened, or ever could happen. "Let one of my children go to New York!" Aline snorts. "Jeez! At eleven! *Never*. My husband would not stand for that."

As Terry and Lorraine moved into their teens, they already seemed a settled couple. They made a good-looking pair – Lorraine so dainty and assured and Terry a muscular, plucky youth. Everyone admired Terry, even the teachers who tutored him after school in order to improve his indifferent marks, and Lorraine was much envied to have the besotted attention of the school sports hero.

Neither had any expectation of going to college or university. If Lorraine thought about her future at all, she expected she would marry someone, maybe Terry, and wind up in a flat much like the ones she had always known in Pointe St-Charles or maybe, if she was lucky, Verdun, a better neighbourhood. Terry had no doubt where he was headed. He bragged everywhere that he would play professional football.

"You are too small for football," his father told him repeatedly. "Are you crazy? They'll kill you." Everyone else said the same. "Oh really?" he would say, his green eyes grim. "Just watch me."

By the time they were seventeen Terry and Lorraine were lovers. The Sisters of the Holy Cross had instilled in Lorraine a deep fear of sex, a specialty for which nuns once were renowned, but Terry said to Lorraine, "Don't be silly." It took her forever to agree, and when she did, it was mostly from fear that a perpetually frustrated Terry would go elsewhere. They had a clumsy time in the beginning, both being virgins, but after the first awkwardness in Lorraine's bedroom after her mother, a heavy sleeper, had gone to bed, quick and furtive intercourse became part of their lives. Contraception was not available to either of them, and Lorraine lived in terror of getting pregnant.

In the summer of 1962, when Terry was eighteen, he finished at D'Arcy McGee high school in Montreal. At the time, J.I. Albrecht was the genial and loquacious director of player personnel for the Montreal Alouettes, which put him in charge of finding Canadian talent for the team. It was his idea to send scouts to watch high school football games all over Ontario and Quebec to spot potential acquisitions, and he also asked high school coaches in the two provinces to give him the names of their best players. The top seventy-two teenagers thus identified would be invited to attend a two-week summer training camp, called the Canadian Camp, so he could look them over with a view to future enlistment.

The names of the chosen seventy-two players were published in Montreal newspapers, both English and French. Terry Evanshen was incredulous that his name was not among them. At his high school he was known as the one-man football team. Outraged, he phoned Albrecht to complain. Albrecht explained that the D'Arcy McGee high school coach hadn't listed him. He prepared to hang up.

"Listen," Terry told him insistently, "I'm better than anyone on that list."

"Your coach didn't think so," Albrecht pointed out mildly.

"He's a jerk," Terry snapped.

"What position do you play?"

"I'm a receiver, and I never fumble."

Albrecht was arrested by the youngster's brashness. He asked Terry his size. "He lied, of course," Albrecht says. He asked how fast he could run. Terry had never been timed but he made up a figure, and said, "Please give me a chance."

On a hunch, Albrecht agreed. In his long career in the game he has had some happy experiences with unwanted players. He told Terry he could come to camp for a one-day trial but that there was equipment for only seventy-two players. Terry would have to bring his own gear. Albrecht then had some explaining to do to Perry Moss, coach of the Alouettes, and his assistant, Leo Cahill. Albrecht said simply, "He's so cocky we have to look at him."

Terry turned up on a Monday morning at the old Jarry Park baseball field in Montreal. Albrecht was not surprised that Terry was smaller than he said he was, at 145 pounds and less than five foot nine, but the eye-opener was that the youngster had vastly underestimated his speed. He could run like a deer, and in the drills he caught everything. Moreover, he was so tough that even huge players backed off tangling with him. Albrecht says, "And he didn't get hurt. He was so resilient he was like rubber. You'd hit him and you'd swear he wouldn't get up, but he would just bounce back." Albrecht kept him, and two weeks later Terry was presented with a trophy as the outstanding player of the camp.

That success led to a football scholarship at Utah State University, an unprecedented award for a Canadian. Terry discovered in Utah for the first time in his lacklustre academic career that he actually was a good student, fascinated by the elements of business administration.

Lorraine had finished high school and was working in the office of the British-based Bowater Corporation of North America. Her sisters provided an appropriate wardrobe of neat blouses and skirts, and her responsibilities included such routine chores as picking up the mail. The highlight of her day came at exactly three o'clock, when she was amused and proud to serve Twinings tea and Peek Freans shortbread on a silver tray to executives, who thanked her with aristocratic solemnity. Bowater paid her forty dollars a week, and Lorraine dutifully turned over thirty dollars of that to her mother. Sometimes she sent Terry the other ten, inside a shoebox full of banana bread and other treats she and her mother made.

Family and friends expected them to marry soon, but how could they? They were too broke even to get engaged. When Terry came home for Christmas, it was her money that took them to the movies and bought the fish and chips afterwards.

Just after Terry finished his second year at Utah, his father fell ill and Terry decided he wouldn't go back to finish his degree. In any case, the Utah football coach was leaving him on the bench more often than Terry could tolerate, and he also resented what he saw as pressure to become a Mormon. Albrecht, keeping an eye on his prodigy, promptly arranged for Terry to go to Maine to play for the Portland Seahawks, a team in the semi-pro Atlantic Coast Conference.

The first impression the Portland team had of the young Canadian was that he was too assured by half. "Throw me the ball ten times in this game and I'll catch it ten times," he announced. So they did, and he did – and held on to it. His philosophy was, as he reconstructs it now, "For you to take the ball from me you have to kill me. That's my ball. You try to take it away and I'll beat the shit out of you."

He was growing – maybe an inch – and packed on about twenty pounds of muscle by working out with weights. To minimize expenses, he lived in the Portland YMCA, and sent money home, although every time he passed up good-looking clothes he wanted for himself it gave him a pang. A few times during the season Lorraine took a holiday from work and went by bus to visit him. She watched him play: he was the smallest man on the field, all right, but also the busiest – a two-way sixty-minute man. What impressed her more was how popular he was with the Seahawks. Terry already was attracting a singular degree of media attention as the Canadian wonder-kid, and in every interview he gave he always had the grace and good sense to praise his teammates.

Sportswriters called him cocky, a word that would be associated with Terry all his playing years. Lorraine has always resented this. "He's a man who says his piece," she explains. "He's just up front, no B.S. He's confident that he can produce, and he works hard to do what he says he'll do."

Jim Trimble, then the Alouette coach, was asked about the fledgling. He said prophetically, "He'll be one of the best flanker backs in Canada."

In 1965, when Terry had just turned twenty-one, he was signed by the Alouettes and assigned number 22. His first start, a game against the Hamilton Tiger-Cats, confirmed his father's warnings. Wearing his single-bar helmet with the chin strap unfastened, a macho style Terry fancied, he was dealt by a lineman what the game calls a "clothesline," a brutal whack across the face from the back of a stiff forearm, thoughtfully reinforced with hard padding. The blow, now illegal, could have taken Terry's head off, but instead knocked out six front teeth and gashed his face so badly that it took thirty-six stitches to close the wounds. He played the next game with a raw face and torn gums, and his chin strap still defiantly unfastened. The Canadian Football League, alarmed that Terry would infect whole teams with this virile madness, quickly passed a rule that chin straps must be fastened.

Terry was a sensation that year, a charismatic player who was a crazy-legs runner, an astonishing pass-receiver, and fearless in the clutch. Crowds loved him, and his teammates had to admire his spunk and his willingness to share the spotlight that fell on him. They took to calling him, in an affectionate way, Pretty Boy, because of his fastidious ways. He would smooth his thick chestnut hair carefully before putting on his helmet, and when he removed the helmet at the end of the game, every hair was still in place.

Terry was still living with his parents. Some of his siblings married young and had departed, at least one of them angrily, so there was more space. He made sure his father attended his games so he could see that Terry wasn't too small for football after all. Terry was exuberantly proud to be in the big league and earning $5,000 a year. Lorraine noted that he was acquiring polish, learning fast from observing the social graces of the Montreal Westmount gentry who circled around players, sniffing testosterone, and a generosity of spirit was emerging that she had not seen before. He spent off-season time performing such good deeds as speaking to youth organizations and playing basketball with hard-luck teenagers in high school gyms. In time Montreal's Knights of Pythius gave him an award as the athlete who had done the most to combat juvenile delinquency.

Lorraine had always thought that it was possible they might go separate ways — she suspected that sometimes Terry cheated on her — but she changed her mind. He has a good heart, she decided. She concluded she was really in love.

At the end of the 1965 season Terry's record was that of the best pass-catcher in the eastern division of the CFL. He was elated to be named Rookie of the Year and, most astonishing for a rookie, he was the football writers' pick for the CFL Eastern Division All-Star team. He received the award at a gala ceremony, which Terry attended in impeccable tailoring. His entire wardrobe was splendid: he discovered that star football players can get extraordinarily good deals from worshipping haberdashers, and he was never shy about asking.

A small bonus went with his awards — Lorraine thinks no more than five hundred dollars, and probably less — but it enabled Terry to pay $175 for an engagement ring with a poignantly tiny diamond. He dropped in unannounced at the flat in LaSalle where Lorraine had moved with her mother, and presented the ring. Lorraine says, "It was hilarious. I was in the grubbiest clothes in the whole wide world, my hair was in rollers, and I think I had a little bit of acne."

As he slipped the ring on her finger, she wept. "How could you even think of giving me this the way I look?" she sobbed. He answered with a disarming grin, "If I can take you like this, I can take you any way."

Lorraine had to laugh. "You've seen me at my worst," she promised.

Terry's next move was to notify the Alouettes that he expected a large raise. The $5,000 had stopped looking like a lot of money, especially when he learned that Americans in the CFL were receiving much, much more. Declaring that he was a better football player, at twenty-two years of age, than any American in the league, he said he wanted to be paid appropriately. He thought $20,000 a season was about right. The Alouettes offered him a five-hundred-dollar raise, which caused Terry to yell.

In a boneheaded decision they long regretted, the Alouettes responded by trading Terry to the Calgary Stampeders, an even swap for a player who didn't last the season. "A super goof," moaned sports writer Ted Blackman. Ralph Golston, defending his trade, retorted that Evanshen's evaluation of himself was "a little out of line."

Terry was appalled and humiliated. Alberta was more foreign to the Montrealer than the States had been. He could not imagine living there, nor could Lorraine. "What the hell did we know of any other *city*, let alone western Canada?" says Lorraine. "All we could think of was cowboys and Indians." Albrecht says that Terry was so infuriated that he chased a terrified coach around his office, and had to be restrained from tearing him apart.

On the bright side, Calgary signed Terry to a three-year contract at $17,000 a season, plus bonus clauses and a one-year option. That made up a lot for the sting of his dismissal from the Alouettes.

Lorraine had been promoted to receptionist at Bowater, and then to teletype operator. When Bowater suddenly folded its Montreal office, she moved seamlessly to an advertising agency in the same building, where she was the receptionist at two hundred dollars a week. But her good job was only part of the reason she was reluctant to move with Terry to Calgary. Her mother was aging and she felt it would be ungrateful of her to leave abruptly. She decided she would remain in Montreal until her mother accustomed herself to the idea that her last child soon would be gone.

Terry's friendliness and zest enabled him to adjust easily to life in Calgary, and he entered into the best years of his football life.

Lorraine says he all but lived at McMahon Stadium. Practices didn't start until three in the afternoon, but Terry arrived at ten in the morning to lift weights by himself and watch films of the next team he would face. Lorraine says that other ballplayers would say, "Are you bloody nuts?" but everything in his life had given Terry the message that he had to work harder than everyone else to get what he wanted.

Terry, wearing number 25, and the gangly long-jawed Calgary quarterback Peter Liske, an American import, practised tirelessly, often the only men on the field, perfecting balletic passing plays. Until darkness fell, they rehearsed the thousand-and-one, thousand-and-two timing count from the snap that enabled Liske, an outstanding hurler, to throw the ball to an empty space on the field and know that Terry would be there when it came down. "My midget receiver," Liske called him fondly. The two men developed an almost intuitive knowledge of one another's moves which provided the country with the sight of football at its graceful best. The pair became overnight CFL legends. One of the thrills of a lifetime for fans was the day Terry scored on a 109-yard run, the full length of the field; only two other players have ever done that. At the end of the 1966 season, Terry was runner-up for the Schenley Award as the league's most outstanding Canadian.

Terry and Lorraine kept in touch by telephone, and two or three times during the season she flew to Calgary to stay with him in a grim basement apartment that they dubbed the Bat Cave. The couple still had no access to contraceptives and Lorraine was both grateful and amazed that she did not become pregnant.

Meanwhile, however, she was rapidly moving up in the advertising agency. Learning on the job with an aptitude that has never left her, she was soon secretary to a top account executive.

By the end of his first year in Calgary, the wildly popular Terry Evanshen was booked for a number of banquet speeches in Alberta during the off-season. He flew to Montreal and told Lorraine that he was not going back to Calgary alone. "We are getting married," he announced. "Right now."

The wedding took place on December 10, 1966, in St. Jean Brebeuf Roman Catholic church in LaSalle. Lorraine's brother walked her down the aisle and Steven Evanshen, the oldest of the Evanshen twelve, was the best man. Lorraine's beloved sister Clare Dozois was the matron of honour. A seamstress made Lorraine a long white dress with simple lines that flattered her small figure. With it she wore a short veil attached to a pert pillbox hat like Jackie Kennedy's, and the final and best touch was a rented white mink shoulder wrap. The reception was at the LaSalle Golf and Country Club, which felt very fancy to them both. The couple invited a hundred people, many of them very large men who played pro football for a living.

Most of the Evanshens attended, not all of them in good humour. Terry was the family's only celebrity and many Evanshens thought he could have done better than marry someone from Pointe St-Charles. Aline didn't enjoy the wedding at all. She felt snubbed by the Galarneaus. "They think they're better than we are," she complained, her back stiff and her brown eyes flashing.

The couple flew to Miami for their honeymoon and stayed in a motel on the beach. Lorraine never gave a thought to the words of her wedding vows: to love and to cherish *in sickness and in health*. She hadn't really been listening and, anyhow, the ominous sound of the injunction didn't jibe with the shining prospects of the young Evanshens. They were both twenty-two.

FIVE

The young couple had been home from Florida little more than a week when they packed their clothes and wedding gifts into a powder-blue Mustang convertible Terry had purchased second-hand, and drove to Calgary. January is not a propitious time to cross the Canadian Prairies by car. "I was petrified," Lorraine says. "I think I cried ten hours a day. We couldn't see for the snow. We just followed the trucks."

They moved into the Bat Cave, with Lorraine already lonely for her mother. Terry, however, was in his element in Calgary, giving speeches at banquets, greeting the fans. Many nights she sat at home alone and weeping, not even knowing where he was.

Their first friends in Calgary were two couples old enough to be their parents. Hal Walker was sports editor of the *Calgary Herald* and an irrepressible football fan who was awed by Terry's talent. He and his new wife, Betty, lived around the corner from the Evanshens. Lorraine and Betty, both of them homesick, formed a friendship that began on the bedrock of their distaste for Calgary.

It was a second marriage for both Betty and Hal. Betty's first husband was the legendary Toronto Maple Leaf goalie Turk Broda. It was a sight at post-war hockey games in the Gardens to watch Betty, a tiny, carefully made-up woman with bright blonde hair, lead her three daughters to their seats, the little girls in matching dresses fit for a birthday party. Hal Walker was a ruddy-faced, good-hearted man who put away one or two bottles of booze a day in the tradition of sports writers of a lustier age.

The other couple who befriended the young Evanshens were Rio and Sonia Sollway, also of an age to be their parents. The Sollways owned the Shirt Shop, and later the Clothes Closet, both meccas for football players looking for discounts. They were the first people Terry took Lorraine to meet. The Sollways, who remain close friends with the Evanshens, took a kindly and parental interest in the couple and did much to ease Lorraine's anguished adjustment to Calgary. "Wonderful people," says Lorraine, and Terry nods emphatically. "Just wonderful people."

Betty Walker says that Terry was the most popular football player in Calgary. "Good speaker, beautiful dresser, lovely smile," she recalls fondly. "And a nice butt." She testifies to the fact that Terry was never a drinker. "He and Peter Liske came over for dinner one night before their wives arrived," she says with an amused chuckle. "For some reason Terry had three beers, and he wasn't used to it. He couldn't handle it. He was crawling on the floor."

The 1967 season in Calgary was another great one for Terry. In one game Terry caught five passes and scored touchdowns on three of them. For the second year he was named to the CFL All-Star team, and he won his first Schenley Award for the league's most outstanding Canadian player. In the Grey Cup semi-final game that year with Saskatchewan on an icy field, Terry's cleats caught on the frozen ground just as he caught a pass from Liske, and two Roughriders tackled him. They went down in a squirming heap, Terry on the bottom, and as a third Roughrider threw himself on top of them, Terry heard his leg snap. Waiting for the stretcher, he begged, "Tell me it isn't broken. Please tell me it isn't broken." But the bone had shattered just above the ankle, and required a pin to hold the pieces together. Weeks later when Terry accepted his Schenley Award he was still in a wheelchair. His surgeon predicted gloomily that he might not ever play again, but as soon as the cast was off Terry started working out five hours a day to strengthen his injured leg, and eight months later he was running at his former speed.

Calgary fans voted Terry their favourite player and presented him with a live steer. Lorraine had the animal butchered and considerately threw a barbecue for the whole team.

Lorraine's mood brightened in the summer of 1967 when the Evanshens moved into a newly constructed downtown apartment building, Charter Towers. They revelled in the newness, the spacious two-bedroom layout, the balcony overlooking the swimming pool, the wall-to-wall carpeting, and an entrance hall walled in customized grey brick. The bonus money from Terry's awards helped pay for the apartment and they filled it with spanking new furniture.

The 1967 season was difficult for Terry because he developed mononucleosis that summer and was wiped out throughout the football season. Even though he could scarcely crawl out of bed, he didn't miss a game. He played at close to his old form by taking injections of B-12 before and during the game to keep him from collapsing. He took to reading Dale Carnegie's *The Power of Positive Thinking* over and over, which he credited with helping him get out on the field despite being crippled with fatigue.

The next year was a devastating one for the Evanshen family. Steven, Terry's oldest brother, died from eating poisonous mushrooms. Terry flew east for the funeral, shocked at the loss of one of the family's brightest and best.

Though the Stampeders made the Grey Cup final in 1968, and Terry scored two touchdowns in the game, he was an unhappy man, quarrelling with management over the usual: his salary. His contract was about to expire and he wanted a new one at $35,000 a year, something unheard of for a Canadian player. "No Canadian is worth that kind of money," he was told.

"Then I'll play in the States," Terry responded.

"Do you think you're good enough?" he was asked.

"I've never doubted that fact," he said calmly.

Shortly afterwards Terry got a feeler from Denver in the National Football League. Just as talks became serious, he received a phone call from Alan Eagleson, the sleazy lawyer-agent who later was forced to give back his Order of Canada, and wound up in jail for stealing from the hockey players he represented. Eagleson had heard about the pending deal and offered to negotiate with Denver on Terry's behalf. Lorraine, who took a dislike to Eagleson in just one phone conversation she had with him, urged Terry to reject the overture.

Eventually Terry turned down the offer to try out with Denver. Neither Evanshen was anxious to leave Canada, but the decision was influenced more strongly by horror stories they heard from teammates about players who went to an NFL camp expecting that they had made the team, but were ruthlessly cut only days later.

Lorraine thought privately that Terry would be "lost in the shuffle" in the States. Albrecht doesn't believe that for a minute. He says Terry would have been the only man in football history to make both the NFL and CFL Halls of Fame.

Prior to the 1969 season, Peter Liske left Calgary to play in the American Football League, and Terry didn't click as well with the Stampeder quarterbacks who succeeded him. Lorraine had a different preoccupation. Though the couple still used no birth control, she was not pregnant. Two and a half years had passed since her wedding with no sign of a baby. Worried, she went to Dr. Tess Truman, a Calgary gynecologist. Eventually Truman prescribed fertility drugs, which worked almost immediately. Terry was in the delivery room in Foothills Hospital on April 30, 1970, when Tracy Lee was born. Advised she had a daughter, Lorraine burst into tears. Certain that Terry wanted a boy, she felt she had failed him. She wailed, "I'm sorry," and he said, "Don't be silly. It's really okay."

He proved it by doting on the infant. When Tracy cried, he walked around the apartment with her in his arms, and fed her a bottle when she was hungry. He took her everywhere to show her off, including football practices. "I love babies," he explained.

Denied the raise he wanted, Terry was looking around for another team as the 1970 season approached. Happily, his friend and staunch admirer Albrecht was back with the Montreal Alouettes and wanted him home. So did Sam Berger, the new owner of the Alouettes, and Sam Etcheverry, the coach. Tracy was one month old when the Alouettes offered Terry a gratifying three-year $100,000 contract plus bonuses and a one-year option clause.

When Terry turned up at training camp in 1970, the Alouettes had a new coach, Jimmy Orr, who had played twelve years in the National Football League. He was astounded by Terry. "There's no doubt in my mind that this kid could make it in the NFL," he declared. "He's quick, and quickness is a bigger asset than just plain speed. . . . And he's got excellent hands."

While in Calgary, Terry had assumed the mortgage payments, hefty property taxes and upkeep expenses for a splendid three-storey mansion in Montreal in which his parents were living with their two youngest sons, Perry and David, both of them still in school. Temporarily flush from a mining deal, John Evanshen had purchased the house on Madison Avenue just off Sherbrooke in Notre-Dame-de-Grâce, a tony neighbourhood always known as N.D.G. The impressive residence had three fireplaces, one of them with a marble surround, and was still equipped with the buzzers once used to summon servants. Though Terry had assumed all the expenses of that house, the ownership was somewhat unclear, so Terry and Lorraine looked elsewhere for a place to live. They rented a sparkling duplex in LaSalle on the St. Lawrence River for a thousand dollars a month.

A few months after they settled in, Lorraine was stricken by the death of her mother. Susie died of pneumonia in 1971 on her seventy-first birthday.

Apart from that tragic loss, the Evanshens were having a fine time. Lorraine was back among her family and old friends, and Terry was playing brilliant football that made the fans delirious.

Their first year in Montreal, 1970, the Alouettes won the Grey Cup against Terry's former team, the Calgary Stampeders. Though Terry failed to score, he played a heady game and it was a sweet victory for him.

Peter Dalla Riva, an Italian-born all-star wide receiver and CFL Hall of Fame member whose number 74 was retired when his fourteen-year Alouette career ended, was Terry's roommate when the team was on the road. He remembers those years fondly. Dalla Riva, now a custom broker in Montreal, looks exactly as a former professional football player should: he is a large, handsome, broken-nosed, well-groomed, fit man with wide shoulders and bulging biceps. After he comes through a revolving door, it spins a while. He says football got him out of Hamilton's steel mills, and he has always felt close to Terry because of the hard poverty they both knew as children.

"Terry played in a big man's game, but he played big," Dalla Riva says with affection. Heterosexual pro athletes, like men who go into combat together, are unafraid to admit openly that they care for one another. "He played the game hard and he had no fear. He's had to prove himself all his life."

Dalla Riva is not only an authority on Terry's courage but he also knows something about the brain damage football players suffered in the days when helmets did not give the players much protection and ignorance of brain physiology was rampant. "You'd come off the field dazed," he explains. "They just gave you some smelling salts and you were back out there again. I'd keep a bottle of smelling salts by the bench until it ran out, and then I'd get a new one. Terry the same. You got used to it."

Terry played four years, the seasons 1970 to 1973, for the Alouettes. In 1971 he won his second Schenley and was

All-Eastern wide receiver. When the time came for his contract to expire, he expected a new one with a raise. At the same time he was agitating for player pensions and complaining that he wasn't being used enough by the new coach, Marv Levy. Management responded to his request for more money by saying that he was almost thirty years old. Terry replied, *So what!* A heated debate ensued. Montreal held firm and so did Terry, so there was no contract, and for a terrifying time Terry dangled.

Jerry Williams, head coach of the Hamilton Tiger-Cats, called one day just before 1974 training camps were due to open. Williams, who had coached Terry in Calgary, wanted Terry to join him in Hamilton for a tryout. "I can't promise that you're going to stay," he cautioned, "but let's give it our best shot."

With Terry's future somewhat uncertain, Lorraine thought it best to remain in Montreal with Tracy, still a toddler. Because Terry's income was not assured, they worried about maintaining two establishments, the expensive duplex in LaSalle and the house on Madison where Terry's parents and brothers still lived. In addition, they had bought, at the extraordinary bargain price of $20,000, a lakefront cottage at Val David, which meant they also had payments on a bank loan to meet. Terry and Lorraine decided they had no choice but to give up the duplex. Lorraine moved with Tracy into a bedroom in the Madison house, storing their furniture ceiling-high in the dining room.

The arrangement was uncomfortable for all of them. Aline beseeched John to move out and let Terry and Lorraine have the house, but he was happy where he was. Finally Aline left, moving in with friends who lived in the country. John took the hint; four months later he too was gone. For about a year, while Perry and Dave finished school, Lorraine was house mother to them.

In 1974 Terry signed a three-year contract, with an option for one year more, with the Hamilton Tiger-Cats at the poisoned end of Lake Ontario. It was agreed that Lorraine should stay in Montreal in the interest of stability for Tracy. Terry's exuberance and love of the game was unbroken. He still went into the huddle with his old pumped-up style. "I'm open, I'm *open*," he would say to the quarterback. "Throw me the ball. We're going to win this game." When Jerry Williams left, however, the plays changed. No one threw him the ball.

Terry suffered his third and last significant football injury while playing for Hamilton. In the pile-up of bodies that ensued when he caught a short pass, three of his ribs were broken. The pain was so excruciating, even for him, that he couldn't straighten. He missed three games, the only games he was out in his whole career, and afterwards played with the benefit of Novocaine injections.

"Half the team played on Novocaine," Lorraine says. "They were all afraid of losing their jobs if they missed too many games, and those football jobs were all they had."

In October of Terry's last season with Hamilton, the Tiger-Cats were playing the Ottawa Rough Riders in Ottawa at a time when Queen Elizabeth II was visiting Canada. A widespread belief exists in the football world that the queen enjoys the game, although there is little evidence that she delights in football any more than she would appreciate a tour of a pinball arcade. However, she found herself one cold October afternoon in 1977 walking along a line of respectful gladiators, helmets in hand, in the quaint Lansdowne Park stadium, inspecting them with her customary lack of interest as though they were decorative posts.

Terry Evanshen stepped forward, extended his hand, and introduced himself. The queen is imperturbable in the face of such unscheduled happenings; she knew full well that somewhere in the stadium a marksman would have his sights trained on Terry's back.

"You're really small," she said pleasantly, "among all these big men."

"Yeah," Terry said with a wide grin. "But I'm the toughest guy on the field." The queen laughed.

With the help of fertility drugs Lorraine conceived again, and on October 23, 1975, Tara Christian was born. Lorraine advised Terry, who was living in Hamilton and playing with the Tiger-Cats at the time of the birth, that he had another daughter. She thought Terry would be disappointed, but he didn't seem to mind. Two years later, unassisted by drugs and assuming she was infertile without them, she was surprised to be pregnant again. Terry was still playing for the Hamilton Tiger-Cats at the time, but was in Toronto on September 8, 1977, taking in a baseball game, when he heard the news that Jennifer Susan was born. When Lorraine spoke to him on the phone, she said, "I'm sorry you didn't get a boy, but that's it, Buster. No more babies."

Terry was depressed, but not about having daughters instead of sons. He was having a quarrelsome year with Hamilton, and spending too much time on the bench for his liking. Hamilton had enough of him, too. Ralph Sazio, the general manager, refused to give him the raise he asked for, so he was a free agent again.

In 1978 Terry signed with the Toronto Argonauts, but the writing was on the wall. The Argo quarterback never threw him a pass, not even when he was in the open. An American, he seemed not to know that the Canadian game has an extra man on the field. Terry managed eleven catches and scored only one touchdown in the eight games he played with the Argonauts, which looks in the score books like a slump, but more accurately reflects his lack of opportunity. Dalla Riva says football is like that. At the end of his career a player can get lucky and click with a team that wants to use him, or he can be unlucky like Terry was and play with the 1978 Argos.

Eight games into the 1978 season, Terry was called into the Argonaut manager's office and told he was through. "Your stuff is in the next room," he was advised curtly. Someone had cleaned out his locker and put his personal belongings in green garbage bags.

This was an ignominious career end for a man who had played his heart out for fourteen seasons, won the Schenley twice, was named six times to Conference All-Star teams and one CFL All-Star team, played in three Grey Cup final and semi-final games, made 666 catches in regular seasons and in the playoffs (the sixth-best total in CFL history), and scored ninety-two touchdowns, ten of them in consecutive games – still a league record. A man who was third in the record book for receiving touchdowns, carried the ball for more than ten thousand yards, also putting him third in the record book, and has his name still among the top three in seventeen of the twenty-six pass-receiving categories in the CFL statistics book. In the list of most touchdown receptions in playoff games, he is still tops.

Terry packed up and drove to Montreal, dropped his luggage inside the front door, and said to Lorraine, "You're not going to believe this, but it's over."

Lorraine, startled, asked, "What's over?"

"Football. The Argos gave me the axe today. Threw my stuff in garbage bags."

Their hope was that his football career was not really over, that another team would want him as a player or, more likely – since he was thirty-five — as a coach. Though there were discussions, there was no a real offer. Terry kept his suffering to himself, but Lorraine had never in her life seen him so depressed. One day she told him, "You know what, it's not the end of the world. You have so much to give. You're going to find your niche, Terry. It might not be today, it might not be tomorrow, but you will."

Terry took his resumé door to door. People in Montreal were thrilled to meet him, but no one offered him a job. It hurt his prospects in language-conscious Quebec that he didn't speak French. A break came finally when CBC television hired him as a football colour commentator, paying about $25,000 a season.

At a Grey Cup celebration in 1981, Terry's second season with the CBC football telecast, he and Lorraine were disconcerted to be told by two or three people that they had heard rumours he was about to be fired. It happened the next day. Vague explanations were given but the real reason seemed to be that Terry was overly qualified for the job. "He was educating people too much," Lorraine says. "Giving a lot of information, and even calling the plays before they happened. It was a real shame they dropped him. People really enjoyed his comments. He was talking to the fans, and they were learning about football. He was very hurt about that." Fans did love him, but coaches and general managers had complained forcefully to the CBC that Terry was quarterbacking every game from the booth.

A few weeks later, in January 1982, Terry's father, John Evanshen, died of a stroke. It happened on his sixty-eighth birthday, minutes after he returned to the Montreal home where he and Aline lived with their son David. Terry and Lorraine had hosted the family celebration, which featured the perogies and other Ukrainian dishes John loved, and they were doing the clean-up when they got news that John was in trouble. Terry drove to the house and found his father unconscious in his bed upstairs. He slung him on his back and carried him out to his car. He and a friend drove his father to a hospital and Terry carried him in, but John never regained consciousness and died soon afterwards.

Though shocked and despondent over his father's death and the loss of a prestigious job, Terry was thinking about his next career. He had an iron in the fire. He and two brothers, Frank and Fred, were planning to set up their own agency, Teleputer, and sell Texas Instruments computers across Canada. At five hundred dollars each, the computers were among the first, if not the first, home computers on the Canadian market. Their marketing strategy was along the lines of a Tupperware party: the brothers would pull together a small group of potential buyers and cheerily demonstrate the product in someone's living room.

The headquarters of Teleputer was Toronto, and Terry told Lorraine he didn't want to live there alone. The couple stored their furniture, rented the Montreal house, and moved into a furnished, three-bedroom apartment in North York for a thousand dollars a month.

Terry, like most of his outgoing family, was a natural salesman. His starting premise was that he had a wonderful product to sell, and this conviction gave wind to his sails, just as his unswerving belief in himself had powered his invincible football career. He had the discipline to work hard, the courage to knock fearlessly on as many doors as it took, and he could make cold calls charmingly. Attractive to women, he was no flirt, and men basked in his renown. The brothers racked up huge sales for Texas Instruments, but despite the Evanshens' successes in Canada, the company was leaking millions in losses and folded in 1984. It cleaned out its inventory by selling the pioneer computers for fifty dollars each.

While working for Texas Instruments, Terry recognized that a computer was little use without a printer and had approached the Toronto office of Epson, makers of fine printers, with the suggestion that Epson throw in with Teleputer. The company was impressed with Terry but turned the deal down. However, when Texas Instruments collapsed, Epson offered him a job as national sales manager. The starting salary was $70,000, with the promise of big bonuses. Terry, Lorraine, and their young daughters moved to a rented house in Scarborough to be closer to the Epson office.

That same year, five years after the Argonauts dumped him so callously, Terry was inducted into the CFL Hall of Fame, the youngest person ever to receive that honour. When Terry received his invitation to the presentation banquet, he saw that it had been issued only to him and Lorraine.

"I want to bring my daughters," he informed the Hall of Fame people.

"We never have children," he was informed. "It's a formal, black-tie dinner."

"Well," said Terry evenly, "I appreciate the honour, but I won't attend without my children. My family means a lot to me. They keep me going and I want them all there."

The Hall of Fame yielded – and children and even grandchildren have been welcome ever since.

J.I. Albrecht attended the lavish banquet in Hamilton at which the inductees were fêted. Each man was instructed to speak no more than seven minutes, time enough to give the traditional ah-shucks responses to their glowing introductions.

Terry was nervous. "I can't do it," he said to Albrecht. "What'll I say?"

"Just be yourself," Albrecht told him.

"I thought you'd say that," Terry replied dryly.

When it came Terry's turn at the microphone, he warned the audience to settle down: he had a lot on his mind. "This is my night," he explained with his customary assurance. With that caveat, he then spent more than half an hour praising football figures he admired (Albrecht, among others) and condemning those he did not (Sazio, among others), even though some of the men he excoriated were in the room. When he finished many did not applaud at all, but others gave him quite an ovation.

"It caused a lot of feathers to be ruffled," Albrecht says serenely.

Epson's president was Maurice Lapalme, who became a close friend. Lapalme kept urging Terry and Lorraine to stop renting and find permanent housing to suit Terry's stature with the firm.

One Sunday morning in fall of 1984, Terry and Lorraine and the girls took a drive along Highway 401, east of Toronto, with the thought in mind that they might see a suitable property for sale. After a few miles Lorraine said, "This is nuts. We'll never find anything on the 401. Take an exit."

The next exit was Harwood and they idly drove north. In the town of Ajax they saw a country market and stopped to find something to eat. In the corner of the market was a real estate booth and they paused to look at photographs of country homes for sale. The one that caught their eye was a classic two-storey century-old stone farmhouse. An alert salesman joined them in a trice and said the property was about a seven-minute drive away. He offered to take them there.

The owners were out so the Evanshens couldn't see inside the house, but they fell in love with the look of the place. The four-bedroom, centre-hall house dates back to either 1851 or 1867 (authorities differ) and stands on a hill overlooking thirty-two acres of rolling fields. The property boasts a green-roofed fourteen-stall horse barn on a stone foundation and an apple orchard of twenty-three trees. The owner was CBC Radio's much-loved announcer Alan Maitland, dubbed "Fireside Al" by Barbara Frum during their many years together on *As It Happens.*

The Evanshens were smitten, but the asking price of $349,000 was too much for their resources. They had some savings and there was the money that would come from the sale of their Montreal house, but it would not be enough. Epson's Maurice Lapalme generously offered to help them out by advancing Terry money against future bonuses.

Terry and Lorraine looked at the house "maybe twenty-five times," Lorraine says, and came to be on very friendly terms with Al and Connie Maitland. With Lapalme's help, Terry and Lorraine figured how much they could afford to pay. With the sale of the huge house on Madison for a shockingly low $169,000 – the real estate market in that predominantly English neighbourhood had plummeted because of anxiety over Quebec separatism – plus the advance from Lapalme and their savings, they could make an offer of no more than $263,500.

Within a few hours the real estate agent said it was a deal. "The Maitlands love you people and they want you to have it," he explained.

The move worked out beautifully even for the children, who were picked up at the end of the driveway every school day by a bus. A bonus was that the Evanshens inherited a barn full of horses who were being boarded by the Maitlands. Al Maitland explained to Terry that barns decay rapidly unless they are being used, and suggested he keep the horses. Besides, boarding fees would be a source of revenue. Terry hired a nearby farmer, Alf Jackson, to take care of the animals and help with other chores well beyond the expertise of a city-raised man.

Tracy was not much excited about the horses in the barn, but Tara and Jennifer were avid to learn to ride. Terry bought them ponies and they joined the Durham Pony Club, where they rapidly became expert equestrians. By the time they lost their ardour for competitive riding some years after their father's accident, they had risen to the Trillium class of competition, which is not for sissies. Lorraine, following them on the pony-club circuit, made warm friends of other horse owners in the neighbourhood.

The Evanshens sank whatever money they could spare into making their home more comfortable. They replaced the ill-fitting windows and doors, and insulated the second "cold kitchen," a space off the spacious main country kitchen with its capacious fireplace, to give them a combination mud room and office. Gradually, one room at a time, Lorraine began to replace wallpaper and repaint the woodwork, filling the house with tasteful antiques, among them two handsome oak ice-boxes converted to serve as cupboards.

Epson decided to expand to include computers as well as print-ers, and took over a company, Computerway, with four or five retail outlets. Terry was moved from the printer division to head the new operation with a salary of $80,000 and responsibility to build the business. Bucking vigorous opposition from the giants IBM and Apple, he found Epson computers much more difficult to sell than its printers had been. In November 1985, he suddenly was fired by his friend, Mo Lapalme. Lorraine, who also was working at Epson in sales and services, was dismissed too.

The explanation was "Performance not satisfactory," and grave accusations of bad faith and malfeasance were made by both sides. Terry sued for wrongful dismissal and many lawyers zealously went to work on both sides of the dispute. In the end, after Terry's accident made it impossible for him to testify on his own behalf, the conflict ended with an out-of-court settlement requiring Terry to repay the advance that had enabled him to buy the farm-house, plus the interest that had accrued on it since the dismissal.

Both Evanshens recovered quickly from that devastating time. Lorraine found a modest part-time job with an oil company in nearby Brooklin and, in January 1986, Terry was hired by CNCP Telecommunications as manager of its western division. He had to take a small cut in salary from his level at Epson, but he was prom-ised generous bonuses. In his first year he was paid a $10,000 bonus and awarded a plaque. CNCP was happy with Terry, but he heard of an opportunity he found irresistible. A tiny London-based company, Micromar International, was making a small ceramic heater that warmed a room with no risk of causing a fire, and retailed for only $139. The company desperately needed a high-profile, proficient salesman. Terry was offered the job of director of marketing at a guaranteed salary of $8,000 a month, plus commissions of one dollar for every unit sold.

He decided to take the job. In February 1987, Terry resigned from CNCP and went to work for Micromar. In the year that followed, his confidence in the product was vindicated as he sold a couple of hundred thousand ceramic heaters to retailers across the country. The promised commissions didn't materialize but Terry understood. He knew the company was small and struggling with cash-flow problems and uncertain suppliers. Still, Terry could afford to install an in-ground swimming pool beside the farmhouse and put a new roof on his garage.

In the late spring of 1988 he was sent to Europe for the most successful selling trip of his life. He came home on Saturday night, July 2, had a great reunion with his family, and went back to work on Monday morning. Somewhere around six o'clock that evening, that life of Terry Evanshen ended forever.

SIX

Horrified that Terry didn't recognize her, Lorraine looked at the nurses in the Oshawa General Hospital ICU station for an explanation. From their faces she saw they were sorry for her.

"That's okay," she said quickly to console them. "It's fine. Just fine. What can I do with him? Could I take him for a little walk?"

A nurse, recovering from her own distress, said, "Whatever you like. When he came around he seemed anxious to get up, and we wanted him up, so we put him in the wheelchair. It's hard to say if he'll be comfortable there for long. Just see how it goes."

Terry listened to the exchange with no show of interest. Lorraine bent to his eye level and said distinctly, "I'm Lorraine. I'm your wife." His vacant, dazed expression didn't change.

She decided to wheel him back to the ICU and she sat beside his wheelchair for a long time, talking to the unresponsive man. "You were in a car accident, and you've been really ill for a long time. You've been sleeping for about two weeks." The word *coma* might upset him, she decided. "It's time you woke up and discovered that there is life around you. I hope this day will be the start of good things for you and for us, your family. And we are all so glad you survived this thing." Terry paid no attention; he seemed groggy, only half awake, a level of consciousness described clinically as little more than a vegetative state.

She stayed with him the rest of the day, appalled at his confusion and indifference. That evening back at the farm, she walked alone through the fields for a long time, deep in grief and asking God to help her get through whatever lay ahead. She felt drained and her chest pained her. In times of acute sorrow, the human heart actually hurts.

The next day, though Terry was still uninterested in her, she brought photographs and settled into a routine not unlike teaching a child to read with flash cards. "This is your family," she said to him. "See Tracy, and there's Tara, and this is Jennifer." Jennifer's face seemed to catch his attention for moment, but not the other photographs of sisters, brothers, parents, his employers, football teammates. They all were strangers. He appeared irritated and looked away.

His state of mind was, at best, semi-conscious. In retrospect he thinks he must have felt confused but he doesn't really know what he was thinking. In a sense, he wasn't there. His brain was not recording anything that he has since been able to retrieve. From his clouded perspective, there was a small woman with him every day, telling him her name was Lorraine and she was his wife. She said he had children but they were away temporarily in Vancouver. Other women came and went – nurses, also with names. Everyone had things to tell him. He drifted back into the safety of sleep.

The small woman showed him pictures and also read him letters. Baffled, he turned away. In time the woman who was his wife, as she kept saying, came with three young girls. She told him these were his daughters, Tracy, Tara, and Jennifer. They wanted to hug him but he pushed them away. *What was going on?* He took no notice of how upset the daughters were. It had nothing to do with him. Then he looked again at the youngest. Something about her seemed to register. He was given her name again, Jennifer. "Gem," he said. "Gemmie." Though he got the name wrong, it was close enough; that small sign of recognition caught all their hearts.

The daughters found it hard to accept that their father looked like his old self, only thinner, but didn't know them. They spoke to him and he responded with some garbled words they couldn't decipher. From his serious expression, it was clear that he believed he was making sense, and the family tried anxiously to communicate by guessing what he meant to say, but they found it was impossible. Terry's face darkened with annoyance. The only physical contact he permitted was with Jennifer, whom he allowed to hold his hand.

His children were alarmed for the future. What if he didn't improve? "How are we going to deal with this?" Tracy wondered, studying her bewildered, angry father. "This is too weird."

He had been a father who showed affection and enthusiasm for each of his children, coaching them in such sports as track, boxing, and football with complete indifference to the fact that his offspring were girls, not boys. He attended every school event that he could, and was an attentive, though often critical, father at the Durham Pony Club shows they entered. He cheered loudest, and demanded the most from them. They were never to quit, he told them over and over, *never*. He expected a lot from his daughters but his emotional tone with them was fond and playful, though he could be strict about house rules such as bedtimes. Of the two parents, he was the more demonstrative, the one more given to kisses and hugs. He used to say to them, "I'm very proud of you. Just do the best you can." It was beyond their comprehension that he now didn't know them, and didn't seem to care. Helpless and aghast, they left as soon as they decently could.

Troubled by their hurt, Lorraine made excuses. His inability to recognize them was because of the head injury, she told her daughters, and he couldn't help that. He had pushed them away because his chest incision hurt. She also had a plausible explanation for his responsiveness to Jennifer: probably it was because hers was the voice on his car phone just before the crash, his last contact with a family member.

Every day, Lorraine put Terry through practice drills to teach him the names of his family, but his attention span was limited and his patience with the exercise almost non-existent. "It was almost like reprogramming him," Lorraine recalls. "I would say, *Look at me. I'm your wife. I'm Lorraine* until he learned who I was. And I did the same with his daughters. He was meeting us all for the first time."

He continued to greet Tara and Tracy with empty stares. Tracy found the lack of acknowledgment of her especially hard to bear. She and her father had enjoyed a deep rapport, a pal-like relationship forged during her first six years when she was the only child. When she was just a toddler he used to take her with him everywhere, even to football practices. Later he taught her to catch a football like a pro. When he returned home from a game, he always went straight to her for a hug and put coins in her piggy bank. "He was like a big kid," she recalls. "Whenever I was with him I had fun. It was playtime." During the year that he was a football television commentator he recruited her to help him memorize numbers and statistics. She would say, "Winnipeg, twenty-four" and he would snap back the name, the position, and whatever he could recall of the player's record. She was proud of her role as what he called his "secretary."

Tracy's most unnerving experience with her transformed father came one day when Lorraine had gone for a coffee and she was left alone with him. She was holding his hand, though he wasn't even looking at her, when a nurse came into the room. He flung Tracy's hand away and turned his attention to the nurse. When Tracy picked up his hand again, he slapped it. The nurse was someone who registered with him, but his eighteen-year-old daughter did not. She ran out of the room crying. In the hall, two nurses smiled at her.

"Your father is getting so much better," one said.

"Yeah, right," Tracy replied curtly. She has little tolerance for platitudes.

After a week or two, Terry came to identify the small, solicitous, ever-present, mothering woman as Lorraine, his wife. The blonde child was Jennifer, and the older, less-blonde child was Tara. But he still didn't know Tracy. Jennifer would bring a photograph of Tracy and hold it before him. "This is Tracy Lee," she would say distinctly. "*Tracy*. She's your daughter. Please try to remember. She's so hurt that you don't know her."

The man Lorraine came to visit every day bore no resemblance, except physically, to the man she had known since childhood. Two weeks after awakening from the coma, he had moved from a vegetative state through minimal consciousness and had arrived at the next stage of recovery, the confusional state, described by such authorities as Dr. Douglas I. Katz, Boston neurologist, as "recovered speech, amnesic, severe attentional deficits, agitated and hypoaroused or labile behaviour." When awake, Terry had two moods: agitation and irritation. He could speak, but he slurred like someone far gone in drunkenness, and most of the sounds he made were babble. When he stood, he swayed and had to be braced so he wouldn't fall. He walked disjointedly, leaning backward and lurching against the nurse, who held him on one side, and Lorraine, who braced him on the other.

He was indifferent to his bodily functions, and messed his bed. Lorraine used the toilet-training techniques that parents employ with toddlers. She coaxed him into the bathroom when she thought he likely was ready, and ran water in the sink to suggest that he urinate. When he performed, she would congratulate him.

To her dismay, Terry was incapable of any of the simple manual tasks he had performed thousands of times. His motor memory was malfunctioning, the part of the brain that without conscious thought carries out such learned tasks as riding a bicycle and fitting fingers and thumb into a glove. He could not wash himself, and even his coordination for feeding himself was inexact, requiring bibs and a washcloth to wipe his face.

"Ugly," is the word Lorraine uses to describe Terry's mood. His finer emotions had vanished. The manners developed during his upbringing in a strict family, his years of moral education as a Roman Catholic, the decency and high sense of social and family responsibility that he had cultivated in himself – all the marks of what had been a courteous, decent man – were gone. What was left to him was only the lowest level of brain function, the crude instincts of rage, fear, and appetite. Terry was as indifferent to the well-being of others as an infant is. He was the sole occupant of his universe. Lorraine, who had loved another Terry Evanshen all her adult life, wondered, *What's going on?*

Though ancient Egyptians and Greeks were intrigued by the mystery of the human brain and offered much conjecture, study in depth is little more than a century old. Early adventurers excitedly (and often wrongly) identified this or that portion as the centre of speech or understanding. Among the earliest pioneers in memory research were two psychiatrists, Carl Wernicke, a German, and Sergei Korsakoff, a Russian, who sought to locate memory by dissecting the brains of alcoholics, who are notoriously forgetful. The memory disorder of longtime alcoholics, their inability to remember yesterday or the day before that, has since been called Korsakoff's psychosis. Fortunately for the researchers, the world has no shortage of dead alcoholics. After many autopsies, both men concluded that memory must somehow be associated with frontal lobes because these were consistently the most deformed in the cadavers they examined.

For a century, brain research had to rely for its insights on examinations of dead brains after certain kinds of invasive surgery or head injuries. In 1830, when ether and chloroform arrived, intrepid doctors started operating on living brains, usually with disastrous results. X-ray technology came along in 1896 but was not much help in mapping the trackless blob of the human brain. Scientists looked instead at certain outcomes. Removal of both temporal lobes to relieve epilepsy, for example, did relieve seizures in many cases, but also wiped out the ability to remember, so neurosurgeons deduced that memory might lie there.

"There is perhaps no department of surgery which is so difficult and at the same time so thankless as is that of the brain," complained Harvey Cushing, a pioneer neurosurgeon in Boston at the turn of the century.

In the First World War doctors observed that brain injuries caused epilepsy, which was an important insight but without much practical application. The battles of the Second World War provided ample examples of brains with localized injuries, and neurologists started to link altered behaviour, especially memory loss, to whatever part of the brain had taken the bullet.

Luria, in *The Man with a Shattered World*, describes a Russian soldier he treated for twenty-five years after the young man was shot in the left side of his head during the 1943 battle for Smolensk. Aggravating the damage his brain suffered, in-flammation developed in the wound. The man lived with his former personality and intelligence intact, but he was illiterate and without any past memory except for fragments of his child-hood. Oddly, he was incapable of understanding the meaning of words and unable to see anything whole. For instance, he could comprehend the tip of a spoon but not its handle, and he could not see the right side of his body at all. Horrible as this was for him, it was immensely helpful to science because the exact location of his injury was known and Luria was able to designate that area as the centre which analyzes and synthesizes visual impressions and word definition.

With the new technologies that permit harmless examina-tion of living brains, the search for memory sites in the brain has become more sophisticated. Abundant knowledge has been gained in recent years through the relatively non-invasive tools of MRI (magnetic resonance imaging), SPECT (single photon emission computer tomography) and PET (positron emission tomography) technology, which enable scientists to see detailed three-dimensional pictures of living brains going about their routine tasks.

The new technology means that scientists can, in a sense, watch a movie of the brain at work. They can see where it lights up when a person is angry (definitely not in the frontal lobes – reasoning power dims dramatically when people rage) and what it does when people are making choices (a lot of frontal lobe activity here). It is generally accepted now that the hippocampus in the temporal lobe of the cerebral cortex is the portal through which information enters the brain. Much of the bombardment of sights, sounds, and data that people receive every waking moment is judged at the recipient's unconscious level to be irrelevant, and therefore doesn't penetrate far and is discarded. Other material, deemed useful, is sent off to storage. But where is the storage? No one knows. And how does the brain get a memory back in order to consciously review it? Another mystery.

Terry's existence after the accident was devoid of almost any capacity for either storage or retrieval. Progress consisted of remembering Lorraine's name after days of prompting, but he knew nothing else about her. The one-dimensional flatland where Terry lived was described by Ken Wilber in his book *The Marriage of Sense and Soul* as a world with "no consciousness, no interiors, no values, no meaning, no depth, and no Divinity."

Every encounter in Terry's shapeless days was without context, so he could not determine whether the person in the room with him was a stranger or his brother.

Dr. Oliver Sacks, the renowned neurologist and author, once characterized conditions such as Terry's as a "state of permanent lostness." Forty-four years of weddings, funerals, celebrations, births, accomplishments, and the inner friendship he had developed with himself, all the reference points that he had carried weightlessly so that he knew every day who he was, did not exist for him any more. He was shown family albums but all the people were foreign to him. In the hope of a click of recognition, Lorraine ran videos for him of family celebrations and himself playing football, but the man he saw in them, the one she said was him, was an uninteresting stranger.

As well, his moral compass was gone. Such concepts as good and evil were beyond his altered comprehension. If people don't know who they were yesterday, how do they know how to behave today? Humans know themselves, their assets and deficits, their skills and limitations, through their accumulated memories. The patterning Terry laid down from early childhood, enforced by his family, school, and religion, and practised until socialized behaviour became automatic, had been wiped out.

His customary fine manners, something the former Terry Evanshen had cultivated in himself, had disappeared. The new Terry Evanshen was without any sense of appreciation or obligation. Despite Lorraine's constant prodding that he thank people, the concept was beyond him. He couldn't figure when "thank you" was supposed to be used, or why.

Since he had no past, he had no sense of continuity with which to imagine his future. He had never existed before, so far as he knew, and therefore he had no starting place from which to construct a new identity. His entire life was the present, which was only a few minutes wide and in any case was devoid of pleasure or significance. Lacking reference points to understand who he was, Terry was unmoored. Everything around him was inexplicable. His struggle to grasp what was going on was too exhausting to be sustained for long. He was alive, but *as what?*

Almost the worst of his losses was the destruction of his sense of humour. Humour is society's glue. Human interchange runs lightly along on a cushion of banter. People communicate goodwill with smiles and comic rejoinders in order to soften encounters which otherwise would might convey ill-feeling. Humour, indeed, is said to be therapeutic; laughing seems to refresh the immune system and hasten healing.

Scientists are fascinated to discover by means of MRI technology that humour has a specific brain location, the right frontal lobe, but a joke is perceived also in the hippocampus, where information enters, and in the thalamus on the right side, which has much to do with sensory perception, and even in the sensorimotor cortex, the muscle control centre – apparently because a laugh or a smile is a muscular activity. Most of those sites in Terry's brain, but particularly the right frontal lobe, seemed impaired: Terry no longer found anything funny.

When awake he was in a state of horror and alarm, but he dreaded the unguarded nature of sleep, and its similarity to the coma from which he had roused to find himself in a strange land without landmarks. His insomnia was extreme. His circadian clock had sprung its wheels; night and day were meaningless concepts. He napped whenever exhaustion overcame him, in short bursts of only two or three hours, during which he thrashed around violently as though in terror. When he wakened, whatever the time, he wanted action – somewhere to go, something happening.

Lorraine adapted to his swings of mood in the mode of the patient mother with a crabby, ungrateful, and demanding toddler. When Terry's wrath flared, she tried distracting him, which sometimes worked, or made soothing sounds, which was far less effective, or else she negotiated. When all else failed, she laid down the law. "Look, I know you are having a very hard time, and this must be very difficult for you, but you can't make a mess of your dinner," she would say firmly. Sometimes her scolding, severe tone worked, like an echo from his childhood when adult women with bossy voices were authority figures.

Doug Waller explained to Lorraine that damage to the frontal lobes of Terry's brain had disrupted his anger controls. Terry had no ability to suppress rage, or moderate it, or direct it harmlessly into vigorous activity or work, as most adults do. None of his tantrums would last long, he assured her, and when they dissipated Terry would forget they had happened. Lorraine could see all that, but would it ever end? Waller said guardedly, maybe. He changed the subject. He told her why Terry was squinting. In the bouncing his brain had taken inside the skull, the oculomotor nerves connecting his eyes to the sight centre at the back of his brain were stretched, but unevenly. The result was that Terry was experiencing double-vision and had to look at people one-eyed in order to focus. This most likely would improve soon, Waller said, when the nerves settled down.

Other odd things happened. When he was coming out of the coma, Terry sometimes mumbled in French, his mother's tongue, which Lorraine had never before heard him speak, and she had known him since they both were twelve years old. When a nurse leaned over him he would slyly try to unbutton her blouse, though the former Terry Evanshen had been almost prim and never crude. His handwriting, once neat, was now an undecipherable scrawl, and he couldn't spell. Except for desserts, he didn't like any of the food he was given.

Soon after Terry recovered consciousness, Lorraine's sister Clare came from Montreal with her husband, Chuck Dozois. Both were stunned by the change in Terry's appearance and his uninterested greeting. Yet, once, when he needed to go to the bathroom and Chuck rose to help steady him, Terry suddenly said, "Thanks, Chuckie." Lorraine, who still had to remind him of her name, was speechless. *How come?* she wondered. And how come he knew the lyrics to some old country-and-western songs? Why did he have these pieces of memory in the midst of so much ruin?

Most confusing of all was that Terry seemed to have little ability to retain information or process a sequence. If he did grasp a simple question such as, "Would you like a drink?" he seemed unable to hold the transaction in his head. When the drink arrived it would surprise him. He might even dispute that he had ever indicated he wanted a drink. Lorraine was beginning to realize that repetition would be the only way to imprint anything in his damaged mind, and daily drills to teach him decorum had a fixed place in her agenda. Eventually he learned to say, "Thanks for coming," when family members were leaving, but he said it by rote, without warmth and with no expression on his face.

The significance of this minor improvement was not immediately appreciated in the chaos of dealing with such an unpredictable man, but Lorraine was the first to realize that Terry could be taught, that indeed he had a bottomless hunger to learn the rules of his altered existence. She derived a measure of comfort from that realization: something of the old Terry was still in there somewhere. The passion for perfection and intolerance of failure that had been his essence seemed to have survived his being blasted out of the Jeep. It was strange to realize that the staggering, thick-tongued, bad-tempered, bandaged lout in the Oshawa General Hospital had ever been a deft, polite, splendidly graceful football hero, but the two persons had something useful in common. Both wanted to excel and both had dogged persistence.

From childhood Terry demanded perfection from himself, and was the most ambitious of the twelve hustling Evanshen children. Bravado was his dominant characteristic. How else to survive in a family of twelve children and a neighbourhood where French-speaking boys set upon English-speaking boys on sight, or were set upon and beaten themselves? This small man had not become an all-star in a big man's game without a swaggering degree of confidence in himself, coupled with a fanatical willingness to work until he dropped. Legends arose about his habit of staying on the field after football practices ended, going over passing plays with the Calgary Stampeder quarterback Peter Liske as winter darkness fell on the field and the cold chilled their bones. In football huddles, Terry used to say, "You give me the ball, that ball is mine. No one will take it away from me." Then the cocky man would have to deliver, and did.

The sports journalist John Robertson once wrote of Terry when he played for Montreal, "The highest accolade one could pay to Alouette wide receiver Terry Evanshen is that he is almost as good as he thinks he is. And that's not too bad when you consider that he has psyched himself into believing that nobody in all of football can go get 'em as well as he can." Another sportswriter noted admiringly, "He'll plunge into the heavy traffic like a snarling bobcat to clear a path to the ball. The key is all-out effort on every play."

J.I. Albrecht once saw Terry in a practice cold-cock a huge Alouette lineman and teammate who was known as "The Hammer" because of his prowess in the martial arts. The Hammer weighed over a hundred pounds more than Terry, and when the astonished athlete climbed to his feet, Terry decked him again. "He was a baby-faced assassin," comments Albrecht admiringly.

This second Terry Evanshen had the same combative drive as the old one. He was nasty, restless, impatient, and ungrateful, but, like the old Terry Evanshen, he was brave and uncomplaining – and he craved instruction. His thirst for self-improvement somehow had survived the wreckage of his brain.

In his early weeks of consciousness, it was this stubbornness that shone through. Despite his agitation, there were moments when Terry seemed to be trying to concentrate and Lorraine could get through the haze. She was beginning to see her future role. She would be teacher-mother-guard. *Wife and partner* would have to wait. All it would take, perhaps, was time and patience. Patience, she knew, would be the major problem for her.

In any case, she was being assured on all sides that it was too soon to worry. Terry's amnesia probably was temporary, doctors and nurses told her, and it was a common phenomenon after such catastrophic injuries. Doug Waller was never wholly optimistic, but he didn't discourage her either. With Terry's diffuse axonal injury and hypoxia impossible to assess certainly with the diagnostic tools he had at hand, Waller could not be sure what lay ahead. He reminded Lorraine that brain injuries are slow to heal. The probable progress was that Terry would mend gradually in stages separated by plateaus where improvement would seem to stop for a while. "It could take fifteen years," he said. "But it could work out all right in the end."

Lorraine's gut feeling was otherwise. She believed that it was never going to be all right. "I just hoped and prayed that I would have the energy and the continued love for him to hang in. But I wasn't sure I could."

Waller diverted her with stories of brain injuries that had resulted in behaviour even more strange than Terry's. Some patients have their memory of sounds intact but not their visual memory. They can't recognize faces, not even their own in a mirror, but voices are immediately identifiable. Some strokes make it imposs-ible for people to understand what they are reading unless they read aloud. Some can't absorb what they are reading unless they sing. Oliver Sacks, then a neurologist at the Albert Einstein College of Medicine, wrote in *The Man Who Mistook His Wife for a Hat* of a brain-damaged man who did exactly that: he reached for his wife and tried to pick her up and put her on his head because he couldn't distinguish people from objects.

Waller conceded that Terry's case was highly unusual, even among this array of eccentric responses to brain injury. The fact that Terry couldn't remember Lorraine didn't have a whole lot of significance yet, but the fact that he couldn't remember "one chunk" of his life was startling. Waller was puzzled. Searching the medical literature, the neurologist could find nothing like it.

Almost ten years later, an account of a similar case emerged. "M.L.," a fit young Toronto man who was hit by a car in 1993 while bicycling, turned up in the neuroscience journal *Brain*, in 1998. His diagnosis was "isolated retrograde amnesia" because he had lost all his past but was able to store new memories, though sluggishly and with flattened emotional tone. This kind of amnesia made so little sense to neurologists — *If he can remember one thing, how come he can't remember another? Isn't memory an indivisible function?* — that such patients once were considered psychiatric cases. The only reasonable conclusion that could be drawn from this seeming contradiction was that M.L.'s brain somehow set up new circuitry to store memories of post-accident events, but could not overcome whatever brutal damage had caused the obliteration of his past.

The team of neuropsychologists who reported on M.L. was led by Dr. Brian Levine, then of the Rotman Research Institute in Toronto. Like Terry, M.L. scored a near-death three on the Glasgow Coma Scale after his accident, and also like Terry, his brain showed little significant damage on a CT scan. M.L.'s coma lasted six days, and when he emerged from it he not only didn't recognize his wife but didn't notice or understand that she was in an advanced state of pregnancy. Much later, under sodium amytal (the so-called truth drug) and with prompting, he could vaguely remember two of five highly emotional experiences of his former life, but not his feelings about them. He soon relearned the practical skills he once had and his memory of everything after the accident seemed to function normally, but his behaviour was strange and he lacked his old warmth.

Terry's damage was much more extensive. His loss of his past was compounded by his inability to store new memories, and his former sociability was not at all in evidence. Clinical neuropsychologists were baffled by the mystery of such vast wreckage, which one of them, Dr. Frank Kenny of Toronto, concluded was almost unprecedented in a living person. Under the respected

Russell classification, Terry scored the highest rating next to the one indicating brain death, as drastic a finding as the Glascow Coma Scale had been.

On July 25, exactly three weeks after the collision, Terry was moved from ICU to a private room on the general surgery floor. His physical condition was progressing well but he still required a second skin graft to cover the open wound on his right arm. On the disturbing side, the amnesia had not lifted one bit.

With the change in location, Terry Evanshen was accessible to a wider range of visitors. Among the first were men with whom Terry had played football. Lorraine, knowing in advance who was coming, prepared Terry before each arrival by reminding him that he used to play football and these men were his teammates. He simply stared at her, as if football was an alien activity. The prospect of unknown visitors seemed to disturb him but he always rose to the occasion by greeting the men with what he imagined to be their names. What came out instead were astonishing bits of free-floating debris in the chaos of his brain. For instance, he called Bernie Faloney, former Hamilton Tiger-Cats quarterback, "XY40," the name of an old football play, and he greeted Heather Ridley, wife of one of his bosses, with "Hi, Classic Coke," for no reason anyone could imagine. When the visitors left, Terry would turn to Lorraine and ask, "Who the hell was that?"

Somewhere in those strange exchanges, Terry began to realize that he wasn't making sense. As long as his circle was limited to nurses, family and a few supportive others such as his business associates, he seemed to believe that his failure to communicate was due to some wilful dullness on their part. It came as an unpleasant shock to realize instead that something was seriously wrong with him.

Most brain-injured people who become conscious of their disabilities will sink into depression and horror, from which it is difficult to retrieve them. Terry certainly had his share of both, but he had some positive qualities as well. His intelligence was still available to him, though scrambled, and there were ample signs that his old determination to succeed had not been destroyed. The mortification that he displayed over mishaps was exactly what the old Terry would have felt, and the coping device he adopted was not unlike the way he used to behave when embarrassed: he started to bluff. Terry began greeting every large man who came into the room with a genial, "Hi, big guy," and it seemed to work. Later they would tell Lorraine delightedly, "He knew me!"

She didn't disillusion them, but she chided her husband. "Swallow your pride," she told him. "It's all right that you can't remember people's names. They know you've been in a very bad accident, and they'll understand. Just tell them that you're glad to see them, but you don't know their names."

Terry took in her advice, but continued to fake it. No one was going to catch him looking foolish. He put what effort he could summon into the task of learning who he had been. He picked up some information when Lorraine read him the letters and cards, which continued to arrive in considerable volume. Some well-wishers were strangers, but Lorraine would fill him in on those she knew. He didn't retain much of what she was saying, but she figured if she repeated the information often enough he might remember, so she kept trying. She told him he had been fourteen seasons in the Canadian Football League, on four teams – Montreal, Calgary, Hamilton, and Toronto – and played on a Grey Cup winner. Apparently that was something good. When he was told that he had broken his leg during a game, he attempted to register that fact, but it slipped away. He learned he had grown up in Pointe St-Charles, adjacent to Montreal. He had no idea what Montreal was.

Terry listened, but he could not put these fragments of information in any chronological order, and it was impossible for him to connect this baffling information to himself. Words such as "football" and "Oshawa" swirled in his head a moment and then disappeared from ken. The concentration required to respond appropriately was exhausting. When fatigue set in, Terry would lapse into distressed incoherence or blank withdrawal.

Despite his limited energy, Terry was driven by his old horror of ridicule and his improvisations became more elaborate. Once he had absorbed the fact that he had been a salesman, which he gleaned from the visits of his former employers, he started telling nurses and therapists that he was planning to return to his old job as a salesman. One therapist even commented on his medical chart that he had "good recall" of his past employment.

Lorraine was being coached by the hospital's therapists. She was told to avoid confusing Terry with too many ideas at once: keep it simple. And she should use the same words each time, because repetition was the key to helping Terry memorize.

In turn, Terry was coming to appreciate Lorraine's loyalty and to accept that she was someone who cared about him. In the jumble of faces he had never seen before, hers was the most consistent, and her voice was the one he came to trust. Nurses noted many nights that he would ask them to phone Lorraine for him and the couple would talk a long while, after which Terry seemed more relaxed.

Daytimes were another matter. His dislike of the hospital was becoming a problem and it grew increasingly difficult to keep him calm. "Want to get going," he kept insisting. "Get me out of here." Lorraine hit on the idea of taking him in a wheelchair to a park across the street from the hospital, and by the end of July this arrangement was a fixed part of the day. Visitors were directed to find him in the park in his wheelchair or sitting on a bench, Lorraine watchfully beside him, while he gratefully took in the summer sunshine and the park's activity.

Soon he wanted to be in the park all the time, but as his ability to walk improved he became hard to control. He would set off, directionless, with Lorraine tagging along and holding his good arm to keep him from toppling. She sat him down one morning and delivered a lecture. "I know you don't like being in the hospital. I understand how you feel about being here. But let me say this. I am happy to take you to the park, but only as long as you don't give me any problems." She was embarrassed to realize she was talking to her forty-four-year-old husband as though he were a small child, but it seemed the only way to make him understand. "If you give me any problems," she went on firmly, "then I won't take you any more."

Once in the park she would help him to a bench and say sternly, "Sit there and don't move. *Don't move.*"

The whole family was learning how to get along with the newly unpredictable, irrational and irascible Terry. One afternoon when thirteen-year-old Tara was with him in the park, he told her earnestly that he was going to buy a golf course on an aircraft carrier. "Fine," she said calmly. "That's good."

Terry was showing increased interest in his former self. When he was told that his father was dead, he listened to Lorraine's description of the funeral and tried to make a memory of that. His mother told him he had eleven brothers and sisters. He was daunted; it would be a while before he learned all their names. He learned that when the accident happened he had just returned from a business trip to Europe, and he tried to commit that piece of information to memory. His daughters rode ponies in competition. He was in the CFL Hall of Fame. He tried to be interested, but it was all forgettable.

Some days he reverted into confusion and lost whatever he had tried to learn. Lorraine would start over, patiently repeating the story in the words she had used the first time. Eventually bits of his history could sometimes make the difficult shunt between his memory collectors into memory storage and out again. Eventually Terry could tell a visitor that he had played on a Grey Cup team. He could not described what the Grey Cup looked like, or the name of his team, or who was on the victorious team, or where the game was played, but still remembering that he had been told he was a Grey Cup winner was a triumph in itself. A genuine triumph.

The Evanshen farmhouse became a way station for relatives visiting for a few days or weeks. Terry's brother Frank and his wife, Molly, went back to Vancouver when Aline, Terry's mother, came for a few weeks, but other siblings took their places and helped out. Lorraine's sister Clare Dozois, a fortress in Lorraine's life, came regularly to fill the freezer with chicken pot pies and other baked goods. Lorraine passed along to them the information about brain injuries that she was gleaning from everywhere – Waller, the nurses, and the therapists.

This didn't satisfy pragmatic Tracy, who didn't want second-hand facts. She talked to the nurses herself and was unimpressed that they insisted her father was making astonishing progress. Tracy didn't think so. She went next to Doug Waller, and the neurologist patiently gave her all the time she wanted. "Just watch out what you ask me," he cautioned her kindly, "because I'll tell you the truth."

"I always knew that Dad would be the best he could be," Tracy says now, "because that was the pit of his being. What I didn't know was if the pit of his being was also gone."

Early in August, Terry's physical condition had improved enough for his doctors to schedule another skin graft over the fasciotomy. The matter was becoming urgent. The open wound, even though it was cleaned three times a day, was oozing green pus. As well, a large piece of glass had begun to surface in his left elbow and would require surgical removal. It was suggested that the plastic surgery should be done at once, but Lorraine had grown fond of Elizabeth Simmons, the plastic surgeon who had performed the first skin graft, and she insisted that it could wait until Simmons returned from vacation.

The subject of Terry's discharge from hospital came up frequently for review, but Doug Waller cautioned against it. He believed that Terry was far too disoriented to be safe outside the hospital. Many nights, nurses found Terry, perplexed and upset, wandering in the hospital corridors after climbing over the raised railings on his bed. As his strength returned, he became more difficult to manage. One night he was so adamant that he would not go back to his bed that the nurses were obliged to make him comfortable in a lounge chair near their station. "Talking frequently in a confused manner," they noted on the chart. Another night, he pulled the dressing off his arm; two days later, he did it again. The next day he was naked in the hall. His nighttime dose of sedation was increased. On the morning of August 3, the day before the plastic surgery was to take place, nurses noted gratefully that the dressing was still on his arm, as though this was something of a miracle. They speculated, in writing, how long the new skin graft would last.

On August 4, Simmons removed the glass fragment from Terry's arm and applied a new graft over the wide wound of the fasciotomy. Finding she had an inadequate stock of spare skin from the first graft, she had to harvest more from Terry's left thigh. To protect against Terry's intolerance of dressings on his damaged arm, she encased it in a whole cast. As a precaution Simmons wrote on the chart: "Constant care if family not available to sit with pt." When the extra staff for "constant care" didn't show up the first night, a hospital orderly was posted by Terry's bed. Later the orderly was replaced by a security guard.

No one wanted to see that new graft ripped out, or doubted that Terry would do it if he could.

Despite the vigilance, Terry managed to tear off the dressing on the thigh where his skin had been scraped. As soon as the bandages were replaced, he tried to pull them off again and had to be restrained. But his cast was resistant to his efforts.

The Oshawa General's rehabilitation expert, Dr. Mark Mason, was visiting Terry daily and had drawn up a program that included gait and balance training and speech therapy. To Mason's consternation, he learned that Lorraine seemed to have retained a private rehabilitation therapist who had different ideas. Mason knew that very little head-injury rehabilitation was available anywhere in Canada at that time, but the plan he had designed for Terry Evanshen was not to be dismissed lightly. Annoyed at what he saw as outside interference, he took his complaint to Doug Waller. Waller, concerned that "vultures were descending" because of Terry's fame and the possibility of a large insurance settlement, mildly suggested to Lorraine that she should not commit herself to another therapist just yet.

Lorraine was in a quandary. She had become involved with the outside rehabilitation expert through the good offices of Terry's brother Frank, a successful businessman living in Vancouver who had numerous contacts with lawyers. When Frank heard of Terry's accident, one of his first thoughts was that the situation called for legal advice. Lorraine and the family would need money to compensate for Terry's inability to earn a living.

Frank made inquiries and was directed to Bernard Gluckstein of Toronto, who is regarded as one of the country's leading experts in personal injury cases involving brain damage, with almost thirty years' experience under his fine leather belt. Gluckstein, a handsome, silver-haired athletic man then in his early fifties, promptly sent a photographer to the police pound, where Terry's battered Jeep was stored, to take pictures of it from every angle. He commissioned an engineer to determine the rate of speed both colliding vehicles were going. Durham police estimated that both speeds had been under the legal limit of eighty kilometres per hour, but the engineer was more precise: Terry had been travelling at a moderate fifty kilometres per hour, he said, and the blue van at seventy kilometres per hour. Other experts were sent to study what in the Jeep had crushed Terry's body and if the Jeep was in any way defective. Gluckstein then made a call to a rehabilitation counsellor, Barbara Baptiste, who a few years earlier had established herself in something new in the automobile injury field – case management from the perspective of the client's needs rather than those of the insurance companies' profits.

A strategy that still prevails in the industry is that insurance company adjusters steer injured people to company-friendly doctors and other therapists, though obvious conflicts of interest are difficult to avoid. For injured people less famous than Terry Evanshen, insurance companies often adapt a mode of denial. If they can, they insist that the person is not injured at all. If that proves untenable, the fallback is to dispute that the person is seriously injured. The final, desperate ploy is to insist that a pain pill and a slap on the back are all that serious injuries require.

Baptiste would not accept referrals from insurance companies; instead, she put her services at the disposal of doctors and lawyers.

Lorraine took a practical approach to the dilemma of having two therapists manage Terry's case: she covered all bets and kept them both.

Barbara Baptiste, a tall, fit, assured woman then in her mid-thirties, headed Rehabilitation Management Incorporation, which is now situated in handsome offices in the banking heart of Toronto. Gluckstein asked her to put together the best therapy package possible to help Terry Evanshen. It would be her responsibility to plan and organize rehabilitation services for him after he returned home, to arrange assessments to measure the extent of his brain damage that could be produced in court, and to design the therapy program that would follow. Gluckstein asked Baptiste to meet with the Evanshens as soon as possible to gauge the situation. She called the farmhouse and Lorraine agreed to take Baptiste to see Terry in his private room on the hospital's surgery wing.

They found him pacing the floor. Misunderstanding Baptiste's credentials, which are impressive but do not include a doctorate, Lorraine said, "Terry, the doctor wants to talk to you."

Terry gave Baptiste a sharp look. "No she doesn't," he said. "She just wants to watch me."

Baptiste thought admiringly, "You're exactly right." She had not expected Terry to make a lot of sense so soon after the accident, so her real intent indeed was to do no more than look him over. Terry's shrewd comment made her realize two things, one of them good and one not. Terry's alertness meant that he was a promising candidate for rehabilitation, which not all brain-injured people are — "slap happy" is an apt description of their state — but his insight also meant that he was headed straight for a major depression as soon as realized the full extent of his limitations, and the probability that he would never be the man he once was.

Neuropsychologists differentiate between self-awareness and self-knowledge. Terry was demonstrating the latter: he knew he was in trouble but he hadn't the faintest idea what to do about it. Self-awareness, on the other hand, implies a sense of self that enables people to go forward with their lives; it is everyone's cupboard of known and practised attributes that makes them confident to consider alternatives and think about tomorrow. Terry had none of that forward view. What attention he could muster was directed at devising a personality that would serve him in the present with a minimum of embarrassing episodes. Planning a future was an unimaginable exercise.

Doug Waller was less than pleased with Barbara Baptiste in the beginning, but later he changed his mind. "She turned out to be a good woman," Waller says. "She did a lot to organize things for Terry. I ended up with a lot of respect for her." Lorraine says gratefully, "She's an absolutely wonderful lady who did anything and everything to make our lives a little easier."

On August 12, Terry was transferred from the general surgery floor to the rehabilitation ward on the Oshawa General's second floor. Therapists there found him drowsy, disoriented and only intermittently co-operative, though his attention span had improved and was measured at about five minutes, normal for a toddler. His ability to identify colours and shapes was better, the therapists felt, though it is known that the brain's colour vision is very vulnerable to oxygen deprivation. Even today no one knows what colours Terry really sees. By this point, he knew all his daughters on sight and sometimes he knew what day it was. Periods of such relative clarity would be followed, however, by a day or two of sleepiness and scrambled responses.

In one session, the occupational therapist asked him, "Do you know where you are?"

Terry replied, "In a golf hospital."

She said, "What city is this."

"Moscow," he said.

"Who is the prime minister of Canada?"

"Brian Donleavy."

"What year is it?"

"1987."

"No, it's 1988."

"Okay," Terry said. "I got it. 1988."

Thirty seconds later when she asked him again what year it was, he said, "1976."

Asked to write his name he spelled it "Terrenccc Evanshenshen."

The therapist said, "I am going to wave goodbye."

Terry responded amiably, "Wave your good wagon."

Another time he informed the therapist that Jennifer "flies her own pony."

Whenever he tired of the therapist's questions, Terry signalled that the session was at an end by pulling his blanket over his head. On several occasions he pretended to be asleep when the therapist came into view. Knowing he was making errors, and watching her record them, was making him rebellious.

But he was building new memories. Out of the blue one day he said, "Tara's the middle girl." He asked Lorraine to comb his hair, the first sign that his former concern for grooming was returning. His toilet training was almost perfected. He could read a sentence or two, if the words were simple. He could follow instructions, so long as they were one-step directions. If the therapist said, "Raise your right hand and then your left," he was confounded and didn't respond, but when command was, "Raise your right hand," he could comprehend.

Presented with a list of commonly used words and asked to find some for foods, he could underline "carrot" and "cookie," but when the test was turned around and he was supposed to name "things we can eat," nothing came to his mind. The concept that "spring" and "fall" were different seasons was beyond him.

An early goal of the therapy was to give Terry a sense of control in the midst of his nightmare. Lorraine provided a calendar and instructed him to keep track of the days by crossing them off every evening. It was a simple tool but he seized upon it gratefully, delighted to be able to tell people what day it was. Another device was a notebook in which he recorded his visitors, and this also appealed strongly to him as something concrete that would inform him what had happened yesterday.

Terry's early moods of confusion and irritation were giving way to long periods of withdrawal and despair. The stress of mastering a foreign environment was telling on his morale. One day he observed sadly, "I have trouble visualizing some words and sentences." And then he fell silent.

His relations with the Oshawa General rehabilitation therapists worsened. Lorraine, waiting for him outside the therapist's office one day, heard him yell at the therapist, "I don't like you!"

Lorraine was convinced that Terry would do better at home, but Waller was alarmed at the burden that she would be assuming. Terry obviously would need constant attention, but there was an additional factor that worried the neurologist. The classic reaction to the kind of head injury Terry had sustained, his loss of control over his temper, meant that it was very likely that Terry would be violent. Waller warned Lorraine that frustration could cause Terry to hit her.

This was almost the worst news Lorraine had heard since the accident. Despite the roughness of Terry's upbringing with a father whose sons feared his wrath, despite the street fights that were common in his boyhood, despite his years of playing a body-contact sport, Terry had never been a violent man at home. "It was not in him," Lorraine says firmly. He once slapped his daughter Tracy's hand to discipline her and she was so shocked that he never did it again. Lorraine and Terry, both strong-minded, had plenty of disputes in their twenty-two years of marriage, and some of those arguments were heated, but it was Terry's way at the height of the fight to leave the room, never to lash out with a blow.

Lorraine was quite certain she would be unable to tolerate physical abuse. She had enough to deal with, she decided, without that. "If he ever loses it and hits me, though I know it would be probably not his fault, he'll end up killing me," she decided bleakly. "Because I will just collapse. I will be totally devastated."

But still, Terry's furious resentment of the hospital and his resistance to the therapy was making life difficult for everyone. The compromise was some trial runs. It was arranged that he receive day passes from the hospital so that he could be driven home for a few hours at a time. The first morning that the car climbed the steep driveway to the house on the hill, Lorraine was sure that Terry realized that he was going home. Once there, he was disoriented but he seemed to know the house. Best of all, he was more relaxed and co-operative than he had been in hospital.

Discharge appeared to be possible but everyone, and especially Lorraine, was concerned about Terry's inability to sleep. Severe and intractable insomnia is linked to damage to certain parts of the brain, and Terry appeared to have that kind of impairment. The day visits to the farm had gone fairly smoothly, but Lorraine knew from the staff on the second floor that Terry's nights were full of activity. He was appearing at the nurses' station around two and three in the morning to announce he was going to the park. "You can't do that," they would say. "Yes, I'm going," he would respond, becoming agitated. "I'm going. I'm going." In the end, a nurse would accompany him across the street. They would walk in the dark quiet of the deserted park until Terry's fit of compulsion eased and he could be coaxed back to bed.

Lorraine resigned herself to the reality that she would not get much sleep. Not for a long time. Maybe not ever again.

Tracy, who was supposed to return in September to a community college where she had been studying marketing, announced that she was staying home instead to help her mother. When a therapist praised her for making the sacrifice, Tracy shrugged off the compliment. It was an easy decision, she explained. "My father is my best friend."

Terry's nurses taught Lorraine how to change the dressings on Terry's thigh where the plastic surgeon had skinned him, and how to care for the long wide wound in his right arm that needed to be cleaned three times a day. With that done, Lorraine stoically declared, "I'm ready."

Waller gave her some pamphlets about a self-help head-injury support group in Durham, and reluctantly agreed to a discharge.

On August 27, 1988, Terry Evanshen went home. Lorraine set the picnic table on the stone patio with her best placemats and Jennifer picked wildflowers for the centrepiece. Terry was a little late, almost two months, but the barbecue was ready and the family ate steaks.

SEVEN

Terry remembers nothing of the two months he spent in hospital following the accident, except for two snapshots that swim in his mind. In one, he sees himself walking in a park with a nurse at night, but the fragment has a dreamlike quality and he doesn't know what he was doing there. The other piece of memory involves himself inert in a hospital bed and watching some people come towards him. They are smiling, but they don't speak and he doesn't know who they are.

He doesn't remember anything of his return home. The new memory he was trying to assemble had painstakingly recorded the faces and names of his immediate family and a few fragments about his past, but everything else from the hospital stay is blank. The memories of pain of his broken body and the massive surgery he underwent are also gone, nor can he recall his emotions when he wakened to a meaningless world.

Most days, the vacuum of his existence didn't frighten him. He had enough to do to manage each minute – figuring out what he was supposed to be doing, trying to understand where he was, apprehensive that he was screwing up again, desperately pretending that he was on top of the situation. The thought of abandoning the arduous, humiliating effort to start his life over, of sinking into the peace of apathy, does not seem to have occurred to him.

His earliest real memory after returning to the farm, the first memory totally his own and not taught to him, is a disconnected splinter. In it, he is walking purposefully down a country road in early autumn with one of his brothers, and he is feeling "really crappy." That's all. If pressed to recall anything else, his eyes fill with misery.

Terry had been home only a short time when Lorraine decided that the Evanshens should thank Oshawa General Hospital for saving Terry's life. Since it would be impossible to find and acknowledge each staff person separately, she hit on the generous idea of giving a party. The hospital provided a lecture room on the main floor and Lorraine issued invitations by telephone and in person, asking every person she knew by name, and appealing to them to invite others she might not know or could have overlooked.

The staff was amazed. Doug Waller says that no one in the history of the hospital, before or since, has made such a gesture. A sizable group gathered one afternoon and Lorraine served catered sandwiches, desserts she made herself, tea, coffee, and soft drinks.

"We would have liked to offer wine," she says, her face amused, "but we decided maybe that wasn't a good idea."

Jim Jack, the paramedic who found Terry looking "blue as jeans" and turned him pink again, introduced himself and the men shook hands. Jack told Terry that he had saved his life. Terry did not seem to comprehend. Jack then told him about watching the game in Regina where Terry broke his leg. Terry said nothing.

"He just nodded and smiled," Jack recalls sympathetically. "I think he does a lot of smiling and nodding."

Angie Bosy, the emergency room nurse who kept the records during the chaotic period when Terry was first admitted, asked him for an autograph which she said was for her son. "Though really," she admitted afterwards, "it was for me."

Terry wrote something that touched her deeply: *To Robbie, Always Try Harder, Terry Evanshen.* The writing was a bit of a scrawl, but the salutation touched her. She thought it was perfect, in view of how hard Terry was trying to recover himself. She has a few other sports autographs but nothing so inspiring. She told Terry he had been just amazing as a football player, and that he had been spectacular when he played with Calgary.

He replied evenly, "I don't remember playing football."

David McKay, the respiratory therapist, was there. "The problem was that we all knew Terry but he didn't know us," McKay says. "He knew the faces he saw were people who helped him, but he didn't know what we did." McKay considered the implications of what he had just said for a moment and then addressed an issue that always troubles people who snatch someone back from death: did they do that person a favour? McKay says sombrely, "Even if we had known the outcome in advance, I still think we made the right decision to keep Terry going."

Marian Timmermans, the emergency room nurse who worked on Terry, said warmly to him, "I'm so glad to see you looking so well. I was a nurse in the emergency room when you came in." He looked at her without understanding, so she switched the topic. "Tell me about your life," she said jokingly. She was sorry immediately that she had been flippant. Terry didn't speak. "The man looked so stricken," she recalls. "He knew he had suffered a great loss, and he was trying so hard to get something back."

Doug Waller, wandering amiably in the crowd, noted how much affection was directed at Lorraine. "At that time Terry's niceness hadn't yet come to the front," Waller says diplomatically. "He was very agitated and restless. But everyone was glad to see Lorraine again, and the girls."

As the time allotted for the reception drew to a close, Lorraine took Terry aside. "You should thank people," she said earnestly, trying to hold his attention. "Just say thank you." Apprehensive that he would begin to ramble and the situation would get out of hand, she said it again. "That's all you have to do," she emphasized. "Just say, thank you. Just, thank you."

Terry raised his arms and the room was quiet. "I don't know how to thank you," he began. He paused and said, uncertainly, "Just, thank you."

Terry doesn't remember the party.

For a long time after his return from the hospital, Terry spent his days in a stupor of depression, a dejected, silent presence with little interest in his surroundings. His daughters were dismayed by his passivity, his gaunt, scarred, and bandaged body, his empty eyes. "He moped around with this woe-is-me expression on his face," says Tracy. "And that was *never* my dad. He was *never* a woe-is-me kind of guy."

Terry seemed to be in a fog. A few times in the night Lorraine had to stop him from urinating in the corner of the bedroom. He hid from any encounter that might expose him to embarrassment. At the sight of a car turning into the driveway, he would run to their bedroom and shut the door, leaving Lorraine to make excuses. She would invite the visitors in for tea and maintain a social exchange for a half hour, or an hour, while Terry waited upstairs for them to leave. She grew tired of inventing explanations for his absence. It was easier just to say, "I am very sorry, but he's not himself today. He can't see people."

For a while Lorraine accepted his withdrawal, knowing that he was still exhausted and healing from the surgery, but after a while his lassitude got on her nerves. She started to scold him. "Don't sit there like a vegetable," she would say. "I know there are certain things you can't do, but there are things you can do and you are going to do them. I am more than happy to help you with some things, but I'm not doing everything for you. There's no way."

She insisted that he learn to shave himself, something all cognizant adult males do without thinking. Terry was clumsy and cut himself so badly that Lorraine was alarmed for his safety. She bought him an electric razor and taught him how to use it. She showed him how to tie his shoelaces, an exercise that exasperated them both. She assigned him small household chores, though it was frustrating for her, a quick-moving, competent woman, to see how long he took to accomplish them.

What bothered Jennifer most in the first weeks of Terry's return home was that her immaculate, fastidious father no longer cared how he looked. He shaved and showered only every other day, and had to be reminded to do that. He seemed never to brush his teeth and he was indifferent about wearing the denture he required after a football tackle. He dressed in mismatched sweat-shirts and pants. She remembers that he went to her school's basketball tournament looking unkempt, which put the eleven-year-old in a state of mingled humiliation and grief. Jennifer believes that his stage of dishevelment lasted a long time, but Lorraine firmly says no. "It was about a week or so. And we never let him go out in public looking messy."

To his family's astonishment, Terry announced one day that he was going back to work soon and therefore needed to drive the car. Despite this burst of enthusiasm, his plan to go to the office proved unrealistic. With Lorraine at his side he turned up one day at the Micromar office and sat in on a discussion of foreign markets, but his bewilderment was evident to all. He gave it a few more tries, but he couldn't follow what others were talking about. The thought that he might be able to call on customers was abandoned.

His insomnia made sleep impossible for Lorraine as well, since he could not be left to wander the house and fields alone. Terry would waken around two or three, turn on all the lights, and insist on going for a walk. His determination was fanatical, and trying to reason with him only made him angry. He would bang on the bedroom doors of his daughters, yelling, "Get up. We're going for a walk."

Lorraine explained again and again that the girls needed their sleep, they had to go to school. Terry would stop the door-banging for a night or two, but would soon be back at it again, and Lorraine would repeat her admonition, word for word. After a while, her determination to protect the girls' sleep filtered into his awareness and he accepted that he should not disturb his daughters. That left only Lorraine to accompany him, since it was unthinkable that Terry should be alone among such dangers as the unfenced swimming pool and nearby highways. Every night,

Lorraine wearily pulled on some clothes and went with him on long walks to protect him from harm.

After a month or two of these nightly excursions, Lorraine had had enough. She is not a woman who can suffer irrational behaviour for long without trying to change it. "She's a strong, strong lady," says her daughter Jennifer approvingly. Lorraine sat Terry down and said, "You know what? We're not doing that any more. I can't go with you walking in the middle of the night and leave three children in the house. What happens if they get up and find us gone? I'll tell you what, Terry, from now on when you want to walk in the night, you'll walk with Rebel."

The Evanshen family still blesses the name of Rebel, a long-haired Bavarian shepherd who was devoted to Terry before the accident and didn't waver in his adoration when his strangely altered master returned from hospital. Rebel always joined Lorraine and Terry on the night walks, and Lorraine noted that the dog kept to Terry's side like the sheep herder he was bred to be. She watched a while and decided that Rebel understood his job was to protect Terry from straying.

Lorraine told Terry about the new arrangement several times a day, using the same words, day after day for two or three weeks. With the weather turning cool, she set out his winter clothes — boots, mitts, parka, scarf, the lot — and showed him where he would find them next to the back door. "From now on when you want to walk in the night, you'll walk with Rebel." Finally Terry understood that Lorraine would not go with him. Instead Rebel walked around the block at Terry's side. "Around the block" in the country means about ten kilometres of concession roads. Each time Lorraine gave the dog parting instructions: "Now Rebel, you watch Daddy, and you bring him home. You take care, and you bring him home."

Eventually Rebel walked Terry in the daytime as well, sometimes twice a day, and always brought him safely back to the kitchen door.

It was a sad day at the Evanshens' in 1995 when that loyal and intelligent animal had a stroke and had to be put down. Terry buried him on a hilltop with a grave marker, MY TRUE FRIEND.

All of Lorraine's powers of persuasion failed, however, when she tried to get Terry to use the upstairs bathroom, not far from their bedroom, rather than go downstairs in the night to the small bathroom on the main floor. Because his balance was so precarious, it meant she would have to get up as well to steady him on the stairs. Sleep deprivation was telling on her nerves, but Terry was adamant about going downstairs and would stiffen if she tried to coax him into the nearer bathroom. "I think that downstairs bathroom was familiar," she explains. "With four women in the house using the upstairs one, he used to shave downstairs and it was, sort of, *his* bathroom."

Terry's older brother Fred came to stay a while at the farm so that Lorraine could leave Terry safely at home when she needed to be out. He arrived just before Terry's discharge and remained for a month or so. Every family has a member whose mishaps become part of the lore, and in the Evanshens that figure of fun is Fred. He is a high-energy, well-intentioned man, but almost too helpful. Noticing the neglected lawn, he volunteered to cut the grass with the family's riding mower. Unfortunately he set the blades too low and skinned off all the newly planted sod around the swimming pool. Lorraine scarcely noticed.

When Terry had been home only a few weeks, a television news crew came to interview him. Don McGowan, a fan from Terry's football days and host of a show on Montreal's CFCF–TV, was prepared to tape a good-news story about Terry's amazing recovery. Instead he found it a challenge to get a single coherent sentence from Terry. Finally he was able to tape a few usable remarks, and viewers of the show were treated to the sight of a man who seemed fully in command of his faculties despite a catastrophic brain injury. But it took the crew almost two days to get that effect.

Barbara Baptiste, the rehabilitation therapist retained by the Evanshens' lawyer, Bernie Gluckstein, became a frequent visitor to the farmhouse. She was organizing appointments with therapists in Toronto whom she hoped would be able to help Terry, and Lorraine usually invited her to stay for dinner. Baptiste remembers one time when Terry, nodding in the direction of some fruit, said, "Pass the football." She picked up the fruit, but that wasn't what he wanted. "I said, *pass the football*," he repeated angrily.

No one ever saw Terry in a reflective moment, simply enjoying the beautiful surroundings of his home. He seemed to require constant activity but his coordination and balance were so poor that he often stumbled and could not maintain a straight line. With practice he found that if he stepped up the pace and swung his arms briskly his equilibrium was better. He gave almost maniacal attention to small tasks that Lorraine assigned. His obsessive fussiness made every activity last a long time. If Lorraine asked him to put a screw into a wall, he took more than a hour to do it while she ached to intervene and do the job herself in a minute flat.

However, the significance of his fitting a screw into the wall far exceeded its practical benefits. Terry was finding in mindless tasks his first sense of peace. He could reduce and simplify his jumbled world to a small space where there was only Terry, a metal screw, and a screwdriver. He tried to make the bliss last forever.

Lorraine understood why he was so deliberate and she commiserated. She says, "It was his way of getting away from us, from the difficulty of getting involved in what was happening. It was just too hard for him to try to communicate." The family dubbed him "the loner."

Most of that period is lost to Terry, but he acknowledges sheepishly that he must have been hellish to live with. Lorraine says that his anger would come out of the blue. His daughters later described what they witnessed in that period. Tracy wrote in a statement Bernie Gluckstein requested: "He gets very upset over little things. He actually explodes. . . . When he gets mad he goes purple, his temple throbs, his jugular goes haywire, his arms start to go."

She described a typical incident, soon after Tracy started a job in a video store in nearby Brooklin. "Dad wanted me to check some prices on a VCR and TV from work. I told him I would get it for him when the price book came in. He asked me two or three times a day, what's the price? Then I got a message at work that he called. I called home. I asked him what he wanted and he couldn't remember."

Terry was hyper-critical of everyone in the family. His daughters stepped around the volcano their father had become as much as they could. Pleasing him seemed impossible. When asked what effect her father's distraught condition had on her, Tracy answers sombrely, "I went from being a bubbly little girl to a quiet and unhappy individual."

Tara's observation is much the same. She speaks of her father's "short fuse." She says, "I asked myself every night before I went to bed why this had happened to my dad and my family. We were good people, and bad things happen only to bad people. Or so it is portrayed. But now I realize that real life is cruel and it's not fair to anyone." She adds, "In reality he's my dad, but in 1988 a stranger walked into our lives."

"I feel a sense of loneliness in my life," agrees Jennifer. "I find myself getting depressed once in a while because I wonder what life would have been like if that man [the driver of the van that hit Terry's Jeep] hadn't changed my family's life forever. My friends think I live a normal life, but they don't have to live in my house day after day."

Terry was easily upset by anything unexpected, something out of place or a routine disturbed. He returned from the hospital with an obsession for fixed routines and permanency, understandable in a man striving to the limit of his ability to learn a new environment. If a habit like meal times was changed, or objects were not in their customary place, he felt sabotaged. The toaster had to be in exactly the same location always or else Terry would lose his bearings and fly apart. He had no resources of humour or perspective to ease the tension. His was the fury of someone betrayed, and his anger brought the whole family running to placate him and reposition the toaster.

Writing sympathetically of another man in this state of mind, author and neurologist Oliver Sacks said, "The world keeps disappearing, losing meaning, vanishing – and he must seek meaning, *make* meaning, in a desperate way . . . He can never stop running, for the breach in memory, in existence, in meaning, is never healed, but has to be bridged, to be 'patched,' every second . . . A man under ceaseless pressure . . . pithed, scooped-out, de-souled . . . It is not memory which is the final 'existential' casualty here . . . but some ultimate capacity for feeling which is gone; and this is the sense in which he is de-souled."

Jennifer says of this period, "The way I coped was to tell myself that the man from before is no longer. But this man *is* my father." She thinks about it. "It really wasn't too difficult. And he was fighting so hard to find out who he was before."

Terry became a clock-watcher, with an unchangeable time for rising and another for meals, though he had no appetite for regular food. He refused to eat what Lorraine cooked for him, not even when she prepared what once were his favourite dishes. His brain was registering every taste, except sweetness, as repulsive. He might try the chicken, but he pushed the rice around with his fork and ignored the vegetables. His wife was alarmed because Terry's weight loss in the hospital had been severe and he was almost gaunt.

The only food he craved was ice cream and chocolates. "Boxes and boxes and boxes of chocolates," says Lorraine sadly. "And ice cream. Like a child. I bought the ice cream in those great big cartons. That's all he ate for almost a year. People who visited him came to know that what he wanted as a present was a box of chocolates."

She considered forcing him to eat a balanced diet but hastily abandoned that notion. She says with a grin, "I thought if I tried to make him eat his dinner, I'd wind up wearing it."   .

His altered taste buds were only part of a constellation of strange traits. Terry's once robust sex drive had vanished. Even his tactile self was gone; the man much given to hugging his family no longer touched them. His diurnal clock was shattered: despite Lorraine's efforts to make his nights sleep-inducing, Terry couldn't sleep more than a few hours at a time. The thermostat in his brain which registers body temperature had been knocked askew: Terry often complained of feeling cold even though his skin felt warm. His colour sense was altered. He put together wardrobe combinations that his family saw as eyesores. For a while even his sense of smell was out of whack. Every aroma, even a cake baking, smelled putrid. (Smell and taste go together, and the olfactory sulci governing both are connected to the frontal lobes.) His balance was improving, but was still so uncertain that even the shallow flagstone steps of the patio were a challenge to navigate.

That fall, Tara and Jennifer both enrolled in a French-immersion school which didn't offer any bussing arrangement, so Lorraine was faced with the necessity that she learn to drive. The insurance company had replaced their demolished Cherokee Jeep with a new black one. She took driving lessons and handily obtained her licence, kicking herself that she hadn't done it sooner. The former Terry Evanshen had been so obliging about driving her wherever she needed to go that she had never given much thought to learning to drive.

Terry was insistent that he wanted to drive the new Jeep, so Lorraine reluctantly surrendered the keys. She was apprehensive as they set off together the first time but she found that he remembered how to drive. She wondered how he could do that, when he had to be taught to shave himself, but nothing about him was making much sense. She was relieved that he drove cautiously, perhaps overly cautiously, well under the speed limit. Behind them was an uproar of honking, which both ignored.

She couldn't let him drive the Jeep unaccompanied because he forgot before he left the driveway where it was he wanted to go, and could not find his way home again. When he wanted to drive somewhere. Lorraine had to drop whatever she was doing and go with him.

Neither of them was comfortable driving in heavy traffic. If Terry needed to be in Toronto for one of his frequent meetings with Bernie Gluckstein, he and Lorraine drove to the nearby GO station, parked the Jeep, and took the commuter train. Lorraine fumed at these outings. To her mind, most of the appointments with Gluckstein were pointless and she suspected him of glorying in Terry's fame. She was not at all taken with his smooth, gregarious, confident manner. Gluckstein, well groomed, lithe, and fit from skiing, golf, and tennis, which he plays with considerable skill, has multiple interests, including sports photography at a professional level, membership on stellar boards of governors, and writing articles in professional journals.

It was all too much glitter for Lorraine. Early in the relationship she persuaded Terry to have their corporate lawyer take over the case, but that arrangement soon fell apart. The new man did not have Gluckstein's experience with personal injuries and obviously was floundering in a sea of regulations, so the Evanshens went back to Gluckstein.

That took them into Toronto frequently, and Lorraine was relieved that most of the appointments at their lawyer's office were being handled by Gluckstein's associate lawyer on the case, Fern Silverman, a warm, direct woman whom Lorraine liked and trusted. The Evanshens were also attending to numerous appointments arranged by Barbara Baptiste with therapists and assessment people. Baptiste was perturbed by Terry's heavy mood of sadness, so some of the work was to determine his emotional state. An assessment in August 1989, for instance, found him "significantly depressed." Terry refused to acknowledge that he was meaningfully impaired in any way. He kept pushing Baptiste to get him ready to return to work, but all the reports and indications Baptiste was receiving suggested that this would not happen in the foreseeable future, if at all. Bernie Gluckstein was keeping a keen eye on these studies. The biggest area of contention with the insurance companies, he knew, would be whether Terry was employable. The dollar amount of compensation would hang on that issue.

The insurance company demanded that Terry be tested for employability and, to Gluckstein's disgust, sent him to a doctor known to provide insurance companies with what they want to hear. As expected, this expert said that Terry had made a remarkable recovery and was in great condition to work. Gluckstein immediately sent Terry to a different set of experts for their opinions.

Dr. George Wilkinson, a clinical psychologist, assessed Terry over several visits. In two attempts to put a simple jigsaw puzzle together in Wilkinson's office, Terry was close to completing it when frustration overtook him. He bitterly took the puzzles apart and started over. Wilkinson concluded there was no way that Terry could work in a competitive environment. He observed, "Terry obviously places very high expectations on himself and when these expectations are not met, he panics."

Wilkinson's opinion was that Terry had no employable skills but he added, compassionately, that Terry should not be discouraged from thinking that eventually he would return to his former occupation in marketing. Without that hope, Terry would be plunged into despair. The psychologist suggested a middle ground, some limited task that Terry could do in his old office that would give him a something positive to raise his self esteem.

Baptiste checked with Terry's former employers to determine if there was a minor role he could play in the firm, some way that he could have a regular "work station" and feel he was making a contribution. The partners gave her request much thought but could think of no task in their small and sinking firm that the altered Terry Evanshen could perform. People in sales have to be able to dance, Baptiste says. They must solve consumer problems, quickly adapt their selling techniques for different situations, show knowledge of the product and the competition, mentally juggle prices and discounts and delivery dates. Terry could no longer do that dance, and probably would never do that dance again.

Baptiste began gently to press Terry to accept more urgent and realistic goals for himself, such as improving his thinking process so he could follow a conversation and say what he intended to say. She soothed him by explaining that he needed to take small steps before he would be ready for the big step of returning to work, and eventually he was resigned to her incremental approach. She kept him busy with therapists to assist in this process and to give him a sense that something was happening on his behalf. He had meetings every few days with physiotherapists, speech therapists, occupational therapists – all the traditional supports for someone with brain damage, and with an independent neurologist as requested by the insurance company.

The family came to dread his return from yet another therapy or assessment session. Tracy comments sadly, "He would be mentally exhausted and irritable, a live wire ready to flare up, and just wiped. He wouldn't be the same afterwards. We kids would just stay clear of him until he settled down. If they only knew how he felt when they were done."

A tempestuous woman like her father, Tara, who was struggling in her adolescence to find her own identity, now says bleakly, "I tried to understand his feelings and tried to put myself into his shoes, but it was hard enough to live in my own shoes, let alone his."

"I feel a sense of fury and anger within myself," Jennifer wrote of that period. "I have trouble sometimes holding in my anger, so I yell out loud but I do this in private." She added with wisdom beyond her years, "I think my father feels a sense of lost love for him. Meaning, he feels that he has disappointed us in some way because he can't be like the father he used to be."

A crushing sadness that his daughters still feel acutely is that their father doesn't remember their childhoods. They were at first incredulous that when they mentioned something that had happened before the accident, he stared at them without comprehension. They found it hard to accept that their new father had never seen them compete in a horse show, had not been at their birthday parties, didn't know what they were talking about when they recalled summers at the lake. The shared history, the fond reminiscences, the key words that trigger the memory of getting lost on a car trip or when balloons floated into trees – the binding of common history that enriches family ties – was meaningless for him. In fact, they could see it made him feel excluded. While he sometimes showed mild interest in listening to the stories, he had nothing to add because he wasn't there. Tracy says, with tears in her eyes, "He doesn't remember us for who we are, but just because we are in his face all the time. He really only met us in the summer of 1988."

The daughters coped by enclosing themselves in private cocoons. Tracy, a small woman who greatly resembles her mother in temperament and appearance, was immersed in her job at the video outlet. Tara and Jennifer went to school, and when they were home, Tara, a stormy, green-eyed replica of her father, and Jennifer, sweet-natured and shy, stayed out of Terry's way as much as they decently could. They absorbed themselves in homework or preparing for horse shows. Lorraine saw a subdued quality in all three daughters that she had not seen before. She thinks that seeing their father's destruction made them confront the fragility of their own lives. Their childhood was over.

Despite the best efforts of very good people over months, over *years*, Terry made almost no progress. He was not even approaching Stage Five of the recovery process after diffuse axonal injury, which is distinguished by improved social interaction and independence. It became clear to Baptiste that Terry would need a higher level of speech and cognitive treatments than he was getting, so Baptiste consulted with the Head Injury Association of Toronto to see what else could be done. That led her to visit Sunnybrook Hospital in northeast Toronto, where the region's most serious cases of brain injury were brought. But the hospital could offer little more than Baptiste already had found. Worse, she confirmed her own experience that there was no residential holistic therapy for people with brain injuries anywhere in Canada. Brain injury programs were only in their infancy, even though the Ontario Head Injury Association, led by Ray Remple, and similar groups in other provinces were vigorously lobbying their governments for services.

For years all Baptiste could do was to keep Terry preoccupied with therapists and hope for a breakthrough. Despite Gluckstein's open-handed approach, and Lorraine's insistence that Terry should have the very best, Baptiste was keeping a wary eye on how much this was costing. The Ontario government at that time allowed a maximum of $25,000 for rehabilitation costs following brain injuries, a sum that did not begin to meet Terry's need. Using actuarial figures, Baptiste calculated the cost of the treatments and supports Terry would require for the rest of his lifetime. Family therapy alone added up to an initial $18,000; cognitive therapy would cost an estimated $6,240 a year, occupational therapy about $5,200 annually, massage therapy $2,600 a year, case management $18,720, a homemaker an additional $5,932.16. Baptiste compassionately listed an additional expense she considered essential to the family's well-being: $686 annually so that Lorraine could take the train to Montreal three or four weekends a year to visit her sister. Terry's rehabilitation costs alone amounted to $45,000 a year.

As the first winter since the accident fell on the land, surrounding the Evanshens' beautiful stone farmhouse with fields of snow, Terry's incendiary temper was keeping his family perpetually tense. He was furiously critical of them all and no one could anticipate what would set him off, though everyone went to great pains to accommodate his testiness. It was no different when they were among strangers. One afternoon Lorraine took Terry on a shopping trip to Longo's, an upscale grocery store. In a narrow aisle near the bagel counter, they passed two teenagers who were having coffee. One of them accidentally spilled some of her drink on Terry. He exploded with anger so out of proportion to the mishap that the startled teenagers nervously laughed, which made him berserk. Lorraine was at first too shocked to respond. Then she recovered and took his arm, tugging him away. Keeping her voice low and calming, she said, "Maybe she did it on purpose, maybe she didn't do it on purpose, but you know what? It doesn't matter. It's done. Just forget it. And you see those clementines over there? They look delicious. Go get a box of them. Jen loves clementines."

Terry turned his attention obediently to the clementines, and the incident was over. Over, and gone for good. The next day he didn't remember that it had happened.

If the clementines hadn't worked, Lorraine would have tried something else. The trick was to placate him with whatever device came to mind, something the girls were learning. Tara and Jennifer went with Terry one day to a sporting goods store, where Terry imagined that a clerk was insulting him. He began to shout and swear at the man, hugely embarrassing his daughters, but both snapped quickly into Lorraine's protective, soothing style. Pulling him away gently, they apologized to the astounded clerk. "Our father has a bit of a temper," Jennifer said. "We're so sorry."

Concerned that Terry was withdrawing deeper into sadness, Baptiste suggested one summer that he make an appearance at an Ontario Head Injury Association golf tournament. Many famous athletes were supporting the fundraiser, among them hockey's Eddie Shack and Darryl Sittler, and Baptiste thought the outing would do Terry good. Lorraine and Baptiste had a hard time convincing Terry to go, but eventually he agreed not only to go, but to say a few words of greeting.

Lorraine says he slept hardly at all during the week leading up to the tournament, but on the appointed day he dressed well, shook hands with a look of assurance, and went to the microphone to say two sentences, along the lines of "I'm Terry Evanshen. Thank you for coming," that he had practised hundreds of times. He got a big round of applause and grinned with pleasure at his accomplishment.

Later that year, 1989, Terry went to a Grey Cup game and was introduced to the crowd. The announcer said, "Here's Terry Evanshen, who was in a serious car accident — and now he's *all better!*" Barbara Baptiste, watching on television, wept at the man's misunderstanding.

She sent Terry that fall to neuropsychologist Dr. Guy Proulx at the prestigious Rotman Research Institute in Toronto. Proulx examined many aspects of Terry's altered existence, including such short-term memory difficulties as an inability to repeat four digits backward, impairment in his fine manual dexterity, word-finding problems, and poor anger control. Looking sympathetically beyond Terry's impairment to the context of his everyday life, Proulx worried about the social isolation that his instability was causing the family. Jennifer no longer wanted her father to attend her basketball games, for instance, because he embarrassed her. He would yell instructions to her at the top of his lungs: *Give her the elbow!* Tara dreaded shopping with him because he so easily misunderstood the clerks' comments and would start to rant. Lorraine was uncomfortable whenever they went to a social gathering together because she never knew when he might explode. Proulx recommended that Lorraine and Terry agree on a signal she could flash him in those social situations whenever his voice became too loud, or he stopped making sense.

Sometimes the signals worked. Too often, they didn't. It was easier on Lorraine's nerves to stay by themselves at home.

Proulx, like many others who were seeing Terry, had only admiration and sympathy for Lorraine. He told Baptiste, "Work with Lorraine. She's his main therapist."

Baptiste knew that already from the hours she was spending at the farmhouse, taking the worried daughters aside in their bedrooms to answer their concerns, soothing Lorraine's despair, and trying to reach Terry in his miasma of hopelessness and rage. She says now, "It was hard. It was incredibly hard. Terry had to struggle just to understand what people were saying to him."

Terry retains little recollection of that period but he has indelible appreciation for the compassion Barbara Baptiste showed him. When he sees her these days, he hugs her and tears come to his eyes.

Most of the many professionals who met the family during this period were concerned about Lorraine's stamina. How long could she continue to deal with a husband who in most aspects was an extremely dependent and volatile child? Divorces and separations are a common result of brain injuries. Couples can stay together through limb amputation, deafness, paralysis, blindness and a host of other bodily disasters, but personality and behaviour change in one of the partners is often a deal-breaker. Baptiste sent in a family mediator, Barry Brown, a social worker with a irrepressible sense of comedy. Terry, humourless since the accident, didn't care much for him and wept with sorrow during the sessions, but Brown was helpful to Lorraine because he made her laugh. Brown's observations of Terry were sympathetic: "His faith in himself is shattered," he wrote in his final report. "His sense of self worth is all but non-existent. He feels defeated and humiliated."

Brown added, "Mrs. Evanshen is overwhelmed and emotionally alone. Due to Mr. Evanshen's unpredictable responses, Mrs. Evanshen has become anxious to the point of being distraught."

Sometimes Lorraine was so tired mentally and physically that she had to stop herself from disliking him. *That's so unfair*, she would scold herself when such thoughts intruded. *Don't think that way.* She believes that a guardian angel helped her get through those lows.

What Lorraine needed most urgently, Barbara Baptiste decided, was to get him out of her hair – to get a break from him. With Baptiste's encouragement, Lorraine one day mustered the nerve to tell Terry he should take the car by himself to do short-distance errands such as picking up dry cleaning. She wrote detailed directions, put them on the seat beside him, and equipped him with a cell phone to use if he got confused.

"Just pull over to the side of the road and give yourself a few minutes to collect your thoughts," she advised him. "If you still don't know where you are, give me a call." She wrote those steps, and her phone number, on a sticker she attached to the sun visor.

Terry often was gone much longer than the distance to his destination warranted but Lorraine didn't want to embarrass him by asking what had happened. Though he never admitted it to her, she guesses that he would get lost and have to stop and ask directions many times. Still she didn't waver in her decision that he had to do this by himself. Her aim was to make him more independent of her, but his absences also gave her temporary relief from the intensity of twenty-four-hour care. She loved Terry, but she cherished the intervals when he was gone.

Two or three times, Lorraine put Terry on a plane for Vancouver where he would visit his brother Frank for a week or ten days. She always took Terry to the gate and asked to speak to the flight attendants. "He has had a very serious brain injury," she would explain. "If he gets excited, just speak to him in a low, calm tone and he'll quiet down." Her last words to Terry would be, "Please, don't cause any problems. Close your eyes. Listen to music. Watch the movie. Don't cause any problems. It's only five hours." Frank would meet his brother at the gate in Vancouver.

Lorraine appreciated these respites but she was growing discouraged because she could see no gains from Terry's weekly therapy sessions. Doug Waller, who had regular appointments with Terry, assured her that she was just too close to the problem. He said he was noting small improvements with every visit, and believed Terry was showing steady progress in diction and coherence. What intrigued him was that Terry was stammering less at each visit. Month by month, his speech was less halting and his ability to find the words he wanted to say was more sure. Terry's brain was making repairs. These gains were nearly invisible to the family because of Terry's stormy personality, but Lorraine took Waller's word for it.

"Terry has that inner core of whatever it is that makes some people special," Waller said. "Some really exceptional internal energy of some sort. That's how he was as a football player — driven, ambitious, but not in a ruthless way, more in a hungry way. That's why Terry got better. He's one of those special people who just have a gift."

It is more than possible that Terry's brain was repairing itself in one or both of two ways. The one, which neuroscientists have observed for many years, is that an injured brain thinks its way around the problem and puts together new routes. Small children who have had one half of their brains removed will nonetheless develop almost normally: the remaining half takes over the tasks usually coordinated by the absent half. With practice, Terry and his brain were learning better balance when he walked, clearer speech, and better recall to help him find his way around the farm and neighbourhood. His sense of taste returned and he began eating full meals.

The other explanation for Terry's minor but significant gains is that his brain was producing new neurons. This is one of the most intriguing lines of inquiry in recent research on brain function. The accepted wisdom among neuroscientists has been that the brain cannot generate new cells, but in the summer of 1999 two biologists at Princeton University, Dr. Elizabeth Gould and Dr. Charles Gross, experimented with the brains of macaque monkeys and observed that thousands of new neurons were forming daily in the simians' cerebral cortex, the outer layer of the brain where learned behaviour is shaped. In a paper published in the respected medical journal *Science* in October, 1999, the scientists described how they injected into the brains of monkeys a chemical that incorporates itself into the new DNA that is formed when cells divide. By this means, they were able to track the growth of a stream of new brain cells that poured into the monkeys' frontal lobes, the executive brain, and also into two other brain areas relating to memory and recognition.

This flatly contradicted the long-held theory that the brain is a finite organ that can devise new routes to get around lesions, but can't regenerate. Much study of the brain starts from the premise that the brain, unlike skin and bone, has cells that can't divide and multiply. In the months following the Princeton research report, scientists all over the world prepared to change their minds. Clinical observation had already cast doubt on the so-called hopeless prognosis following brain-cell death. People less damaged than Terry were making measurable recoveries that suggested that something more than new circuitry was happening: some observers had been speculating that maybe it was cell growth, a revolutionary idea. One enchanting experiment at Rockefeller University showed indisputably that adult canaries grow neurons to learn new songs. Chickadees also were shown to have neural development that enabled them to find where they had hidden food. As early as 1965 several other scientists were reporting that the hippocampus, the doorway of the brain's memory, appeared capable of some self-renewal. The same Elizabeth Gould who worked with the macaque monkeys discovered three years earlier that tree shrews and marmoset monkeys produced new cells in their hippocampi, and subsequent research in Sweden demonstrated that the same cell growth happened in the hippocampus of humans.

"It's a whole new ball game," one scientist declared.

Nicholas Wade, writing in *The New York Times*, quoted Dr. Ronald D.G. McKay of the National Institutes of Health, who has spent years studying brain-stem cells. McKay said that if the brain indeed can produce new neurons in those areas observed by the Princeton experiments, it will have great impact on the treatment of elderly and damaged brains. These are the places in the brain, McKay noted, that are "involved in the highest level of personality: it's the frontal cortex that is important in determining who are you in a very human way."

No one was saying that these fresh-hatched neurons would restore such a profound loss as the first forty-four years of Terry's life or reverse the losses of Alzheimer's disease. While fresh neurons are unlikely to patch up the mess of amnesia or dementia, possibly they can ameliorate some other conditions. New neurons may have enabled Terry to make the gains that Waller noted.

The family's savings ran out soon after Terry's return home, and Lorraine's financial problems became acute. Terry's monthly salary of $8,000 plus commissions had stopped when he was injured, and it was clear that he would not be returning to his job, or any job. The Micromar partners made a sympathetic one-time payment of $5,000 to Lorraine, but that was all the company seemed to be able to afford, and Micromar had no disability benefit package for its employees. The company was having problems of its own because of cash flow troubles and difficulties obtaining parts, so there appeared little likelihood that Terry would ever be paid the commissions owed him from the European sales trip. Then, six months after Terry's accident, the firm went bankrupt.

Lorraine was drowning in debt. She took a hard look at the books and discovered that boarding horses, which the Evanshens had believed was revenue-producing, actually cost them money. She gave the owners several months' notice and moved them out. That reduced the stable to the four horses they owned themselves.

When Lorraine asked Bernie Gluckstein when she could expect a settlement from the insurance company of the man whose car struck Terry, he explained that motor-vehicle accidents involving serious injuries can take five years to go to court, and even longer. Terry's case would not be settled until careful assessments were done to establish the extent of his disability, a calculation made of his future lost earnings, the financial total determined, and completion of what would be a long negotiation with the two insurance companies involved. Daryl Pertan, driver of the van that hit Terry, had a policy with a $500,000 limit, and Terry's policy had a clause for $1 million covering uninsured-driver accidents. Terry's insurance might apply in this case because of the inadequacy of the other driver's coverage, though there was some controversy about whether two insurance payments could be stacked. If they could, the potential compensation was $1.5 million, but Gluckstein decided to aim at $2 million. All of that would come from automobile insurance. He already had determined that no other source of compensation was available, since neither the Jeep nor the van were defective in any way and the condition of the road was faultless.

Gluckstein received an offer from Pertan's insurance company. Elated by the favourable report from its tame expert, it offered a settlement of $100,000. The lawyer recommended that Lorraine turn this down, which she did. Gluckstein was careful not to be too optimistic and raise Lorraine's hopes of a $2-million payout, but $100,000 was a ridiculous offer. Meanwhile, he would see what could be done about obtaining advance payments from the insurance companies. Subsequently, he was able to wrest a sum enough to protect the Evanshens from insolvency.

Practising this kind of law takes steady nerves. If the case went to trial, a judge might not see fit to require the insurance company to pay Gluckstein's disbursements – those payments he was making to private investigators, and fees and commitments he was making to doctors and neuropsychologists. Gluckstein has sometimes laid out more than $100,000 in disbursements in advance of the case being heard. The fee for his time and expert-ise, however, would be calculated on a sliding scale, not to exceed twenty percent of whatever money Terry was awarded, so it was a gamble. At any one time Gluckstein's firm of eight lawyers, one of them his son, might be handling three hundred cases of catastrophic injury and not be certain they would make a cent on some of them.

Lorraine went to her bank, a branch of the Canadian Imperial Bank of Commerce, where a sympathetic manager, Emily Sneider, authorized a line of credit. Their agreement was that Lorraine would pay the debt down whenever her lawyer could wring an interim payment from the insurance company. Relieved she was no longer facing financial catastrophe, Lorraine decided not to rein in the family's customary expenditures. They would not scrimp in mean ways to get through the crisis. "That man who did this to Terry took away enough from us," she vowed. "He's not going to take away our quality of life too." But still, there were times when cash-flow difficulties required her to be frugal for a few weeks or months.

On top of her financial worries, Lorraine could take little comfort from Terry's prognosis. Rehabilitation for head-injured people was in its infancy in Canada. Terry was making some small gains, but his temper and memory problems were untouched by all of Baptiste's best efforts. One of her referrals, for instance, was to a speech-language pathologist, Bina Maser, who saw Terry twice a week and helped him with conversation skills and his tendency to slur his words when he was tired, the improvements that Doug Waller was noting. It was helpful progress but far from the breakthrough the Evanshen family needed.

Money for the therapy was coming from authorizations by Terry's insurance company, which had limited provision for rehabilitation expenses. The paper work, done by Baptiste, was staggering.

Baptiste's main advice to Lorraine was to avoid agitating Terry. Like Waller, she realized the new Terry might well become violent when crossed.

Lorraine had expected to collapse in a sobbing heap if Terry ever hurt her physically, but when the blows came she kept her head. The first incident happened one afternoon when Terry was in a blind rage about something, and suddenly slapped her across the face. She was frightened, since he is almost a foot taller than she is and much stronger, but she responded indignantly.

"Don't you *ever* do that to me again," she blazed at him. "You never hit me before and you are not going to hit me now. I know you have a lot to deal with, and I know everything isn't right up there, and I realize that hitting me has to do with the head injury. But I don't deserve it. You are going to find another way to take out your frustration. You are not going to take out your frustration on me or on your children. Forget it."

A few weeks later they were sitting in the den watching television when something annoyed him. He grabbed her foot and twisted it hard, telling her he intended to break her leg. Lorraine didn't cry out with pain. Instead she said with contempt, "Big man! Are you happy about what you just did? I'm having a tough enough time taking care of you, so now who's going to take care of you if you break my ankle and I'm in a cast? *Use your skull.* I know it's not up to par, but it isn't going to help anything if you hurt me. Go squeeze something outside if you need to squeeze something, but don't take it out on me. I didn't do anything."

That put an end to the physical abuse, except for a distressing moment months later when the family was in Toronto's Pearson airport, preparing to fly to the Caribbean for a winter vacation. Tracy can't recall what provoked the outburst, but suddenly her father viciously kicked her foot. She cried, and Lorraine intervened, urgently pulling him away for a private talk. "I don't know what Mom said," Tracy says, "but it never happened again."

Those three incidents were the only times Terry lashed out, a remarkable restraint for a strong, easily inflamed man whose anger controls were crippled. But Terry, confused and angry as he was, somehow registered Lorraine's threat to leave him if he ever struck their daughter again. "He was not going to abuse his children," she says, "and I made it clear to him that I would be gone if it happened again. They had enough to deal with, without getting hit."

Lorraine noted that her daughters had become somewhat afraid of their father, and that they tried as tactfully as possible to avoid encountering him. She decided that part of the problem was that Terry wasn't showing the girls any love. She talked to him about this. "Look," she repeated earnestly, "they're just children. They don't know what your next reaction is going to be. I could be wrong, but I think they are a little bit scared of you. So for God's sake, Terry, show them some affection. Give them a hug, the way you used to. You have to make an effort." Terry burst into tears. *Hug* was a word he didn't know.

She demonstrated what a hug was, and Terry tried to imitate it. He advanced on his startled daughters, extended his arms, and bent his elbows to embrace them stiffly. The effort was laudable, but Lorraine sadly noted that the girls were not impressed.

"It was a cold, cold hug, not cheek to cheek," Lorraine comments wryly, "but he thought he was doing a grand job."

She reminded him daily of the need to show affection for his children. "Did you hug the girls today?" she would inquire.

"I don't remember," he usually responded. "Maybe not."

"They'll be home from school in a few minutes," Lorraine would say. "How about you staying here in the kitchen, and when they come through the door you give them a hug the way you used to. If it's the second time today, what a bonus." And Terry, clumsy but game, would stand inside the kitchen door with his arms stiffly extended.

As for her own needs for affection, she took a pass. They still slept in the same bed but only because Lorraine felt a need to watch over him. Terry showed not the slightest interest in her. He never touched her, and when she embraced him he merely endured the intimacy.

She says she was far too exhausted to wish back his virile sex drive. "The best times for me were when I got him to bed and asleep, and hoped he'd stay there. I would come downstairs and make myself a cup of tea. And sit by myself. After about fifteen minutes of peace, I'd go up to bed, but he'd be getting up for something."

The girls asked their mother how long this would go on. Would they ever get their father back? "We just have to take every day at a time," she would tell them. "Just say a little prayer and hope he's going to get better. But I can't promise you that he's going to get lots and lots better. We'll just wait and see."

Jennifer and Tara are close, having formed an early liaison that came of being the two youngest and only two years apart. When Jennifer was small, she was so shy that she couldn't speak in class. Whenever her teacher needed a response from her, Tara would be summoned from another classroom and Jennifer would whisper the answer in her ear.

Tara's assertive nature and Jennifer's timidity created a symbiotic relationship that worked for them both, but the real glue in their lives has been the athleticism inherited from Terry, which he nurtured in them from the time they were tots. They were known as tomboys, because of Terry's insistent coaching in rugby, basketball, baseball, and hockey. Tracy wasn't able to be active athletically because she proved to have bad knees, but she turned out to coach such games as rugby instead.

Terry had not seemed to notice that his children were girls. When they started school he told them all that if anyone bothered them they were to fight back, and he meant fists. "If anyone hits you, just punch back. I'll deal with the principal," he advised them. "Just don't ever back down from a bully."

Terry took the view that his daughters were so extraordinary that they were capable of tasks usually reserved for large men. Jennifer, at ten, was expected to help clean horse stalls every morning and push a fifty-pound wooden wheelbarrow. Tara remembers that her father used to take her to a gym where he coached boxers, and he would put her on a slant board and instruct her to do sit-ups to amuse herself. At age six, she could do one hundred sit-ups.

"He put a lot of pressure on us," says Jennifer, a lovely blonde woman with eyes as brown as chocolate. "You always had to try your best, and sometimes your best wasn't good enough." Tara, also a beauty, but small and fierce with her father's electricity and determination, would weep with frustration when her riding skills in pony shows failed to meet Terry's approval. "When I didn't win, he was totally on my case," she says. She adds with a dismissive shrug, "I don't know if that made me stronger or not."

In the face of their father's altered personality, Tara and Jennifer clung together for comfort. The household around them was too tumultuous for either of them to get much attention, with relatives coming and going, their mother engrossed in reprogramming their father, and their father an explosive man. When Tara had her first menstrual period, it was six months before she found quiet private time to tell her mother. The girls slowly came to the conclusion, as expressed by Jennifer, that "the man we knew before is no longer. This new man is our father. We better get used to it."

Lorraine's pride does not permit her to let her guard down except with good friends – "She's a closet crier," says her daughter Tracy – but many times she wondered how long she could stand the role that had been thrust upon her. The problem was the lack of alternatives for Terry. No one seemed to know of a residential treatment centre. She was trapped. So far as she knew, there was her – or nothing.

Barbara Baptiste suggested that Lorraine and Terry attend a meeting of the Durham Head Injury Association in her area. "You might find support there from people going through something the same," she told them. Lorraine took Terry to gatherings several times, but she found little comfort in the sessions. Though some head-injured people had appalling difficulties with speech or mobility or both, and some had degrees of short-term memory loss or patches of amnesia, no one had Terry's combination of extreme memory disabilities and good physical competence. "He just didn't fit," Lorraine says.

In November of the year of the accident, Terry heard that there was a dinner planned for new inductees to the CFL Hall of

Fame. To Lorraine's dismay, he insisted he wanted to attend. The family ordered a table and off they went, daughters and all. Terry clearly regretted his decision as soon as they entered the press of people having pre-dinner cocktails. Dozens of people came to greet him, and he could not recognize anyone.

"He was lost," says Lorraine compassionately. "People wanted to talk to him about old times, but he didn't know what they were talking about. He would just nod, and smile, and excuse himself to go to the bathroom. He must have gone to the bathroom that night about forty times, to get away from making conversation."

Jennifer remembers that few people at that dinner had any idea that there was anything wrong with Terry Evanshen. He looked exactly like his old self: Terry was a handsome sight that night. Friends came up to say, "Howya doing," and "You look great," and all he had to do to complete the illusion of normalcy was smile and say, "Hi." Afterwards he would whisper to Lorraine, who never left his side, "Who the hell was that?"

As Christmas approached, Lorraine was exhausted and the daughters seemed depressed. Lorraine is a sun-lover and looks great when tanned, so she decided that the family's morale needed the boost of a winter vacation in the Caribbean. Doug Ridley, one of the partners in Terry's former firm and a frequent visitor at the farm with his wife, Heather, said they wanted to get away too. On the last day of 1988, the Evanshens and Ridleys flew to the Dominican Republic.

The group was so weary when they arrived that they passed on New Year's Eve celebrations and went to bed early, but the next day they were at the beach and wading blissfully into a warm turquoise ocean. Terry, always a strong and capable swimmer, walked up to his hips, and then his chin, and then he disappeared. As he tells it, and the memory has stayed with him, he was unafraid to find himself underwater. Instead he opened his eyes and gazed around with interest. For the first time in his new life he was relaxed and at peace. Then Doug Ridley, who was closest to him in the surf, pulled him up into the air.

This incident is strange for two reasons. The first is that swimming comes close to being instinctive in humans, almost in the category of the ability to walk. Once people have become even slightly proficient in the water they will be able to stay afloat all their lives. Even non-swimmers who find themselves in deep water will make flailing motions that are not entirely ineffective. But Terry, a superbly coordinated athlete, had lost the skill and would have drowned serenely without a struggle.

His passivity is the second oddity. The pleasure he felt underwater was that of four-month-old infants introduced to swimming lessons. They do not panic when submerged but are content, as if they are re-experiencing the amniotic fluid they recently left. Submerged babies – and the submerged Terry Evanshen – revert to a fetal stage. They simply stop breathing and drift loosely in perfect comfort. Floating beneath the surface of a warm, salty sea, Terry experienced wholeness. For the first time since the accident, he was a happy man.

EIGHT

The Evanshen family remembers the first three years after Terry's accident as a time of unmitigated misery. Terry says of this period, "Nothing was sinking in. I could see next to no good, so everything was bad. I had to search and search to find something good going on. Trying to find something good was how I tried to keep my mind from thinking that things were really shitty. I felt useless. *What am I good for?* I was angry like a son-of-a-gun."

Terry's obsessiveness and explosive temper kept the tension level high in the isolated farmhouse. "You never knew what to expect," Lorraine says. "He was having tantrums, hollering all the time. Taking all the dishes out of the cupboard to arrange them because something was out of place. And you were never sure he wouldn't throw something."

Her patience was not unlimited. Many times when she heard him moving dishes and glasses around, she would join him in the kitchen and say, "You've got to bloody well be kidding, eh? Leave the stupid glasses alone." Sometimes he would stop; most often, he paid her no attention.

Vehemently critical of his wife and children, he was obsessed with order. He says himself that he "created arguments." It bothered him if a placemat wasn't square with the edge of the table, or if a laundry basket was left in the upstairs hallway, or if petals from a bouquet had fallen on the floor. If the cats were in his way, he kicked them. If a daughter did up one buckle of her backpack but not the other, he immediately, urgently, fastened the loose strap. When he got out of bed to go to the bathroom at night, he first turned around and smoothed his side of the sheet and blankets. To Lorraine's increasing irritation, he made minute adjustments of table settings or the ornaments on a fireplace mantel to fit some ideal of perfection that he carried in his anxious head. These changes were not done idly, as people absentmindedly straighten lampshades, but with a compulsion that revealed how Terry's intimate sense of safety depended on an orderly, predictable environment. If the curtains hung evenly, his world was secure; if they were carelessly draped, he was uneasy. Any dislocation in his household signified to his troubled mind the possibility of imminent, unimaginable chaos. When he moved a sofa pillow two inches to the right, where he thought it belonged, Terry was truing his own alignment.

"I would set the table, and think that it looked very nice," Lorraine says, "and Terry would move a candlestick. Just a tiny bit, a really insignificant bit."

Lorraine thought, often, that she needed to leave or "go off my rocker." With a grin that uses her whole face, she says, "If someone had given me an apple and a road map, I'd've been gone." But she couldn't abandon him; he hadn't asked for this.

Barry Brown, a social worker and family mediator in Toronto, came to the farm to see what he could do to help. His estimate of the damage to the Evanshens' relationships was a sorrowful one. He wrote that Terry "feels a deep and profound despondency in light of not only his losses but those of his wife and children. The cohesive and caring family unit that had been present prior to his accident has all but totally eroded. . . . He remains somewhat emotionally isolated despite his heartfelt efforts to again be more significantly emotionally linked to his family."

About Lorraine, he added, "Her friend and husband, in too many ways, no longer exists. . . . Mrs. Evanshen is left with a disabled dependent. By all accounts, the emotional relationship shared by Mr. and Mrs. Evanshen was profound, fulfilling and central to both. The loss of this relationship has proven devastating for Mrs. Evanshen. . . . She is very much emotionally alone and isolated."

Lorraine blurted out the root of her anguish. "It's not Terry," she told Brown, her face twisted and eyes full of tears. Someone else had moved into her beloved husband's body and was using his voice. She was required to support and soothe an angry, demanding stranger who only looked like Terry. She confessed she had lost all hope that he would ever again be the "thinking and communicative" partner she had known. Brown suggested that Lorraine should get away from Terry periodically, especially in the winter when weather kept them housebound, in order to calm herself and regain what he sympathetically described as her "much needed emotional strength."

Barbara Baptiste, the rehabilitation coordinator, was saying the same thing. She kept urging Lorraine to give herself a break. Finally Lorraine agreed and planned a weekend at Val David, in the Laurentians northeast of Montreal, at a cottage that belonged to

Clare and Chuck Dozois. Lorraine left prepared meals in the freezer and put Aline, Terry's mother, in charge of the household. She told Terry repeatedly that she would be gone only two nights and that he would be fine. On a Saturday morning she took a train to Montreal and was driven to the cottage. Minutes after she arrived the phone rang and it was Terry. Weeping inconsolably, he begged her to return. She reminded him that she would be gone only two nights and would be home on Monday noon, only a day and a half away. Terry wasn't mollified and continued to be so wildly upset that his cries could be heard through the telephone connection by everyone in the cottage. Chuck offered to drive Lorraine back that minute, but Lorraine decided she was going to stay.

That night she was sleepless with remorse and worry, but when she called home the next morning Aline reported that Terry seemed fine. Lorraine stayed another day as she had planned, and when she returned home she found Terry indifferent. He couldn't remember that he had called her.

The ordeal took so much out of her that she never tried another overnight getaway. Instead she gave herself small inter-ludes when she would drive to nearby Cullen Gardens, a beauti-fully landscaped tourist attraction, and walk around for a while among the lush flower beds, or she would simply park on a quiet country road for fifteen minutes and soak up the peacefulness.

The Evanshens could see little progress in Terry's erratic, stormy condition, but Doug Waller, the neurologist who had become a family friend, maintained that positive things were hap-pening. Every few weeks, late in the day, his last appointment, Terry would visit Waller in his office atop an Oshawa clinic that has seventy-three physician partners, the largest clinic in the country. Waller and Terry would chat, sometimes for a couple of hours without either of them noticing the time. Waller was soothing and reassuring. He told Terry to accept that his recovery would be slow, and that he should take each day, each hour, one at a time.

Terry was warmed by Waller's kindness and, in turn, the neurologist was fascinated to witness progress in his severely damaged patient. Waller noted that Terry's periods of coherence were growing longer. Though he could volunteer nothing spontaneously he was beginning to be able, when asked, to relate such family news as how well the girls were doing at horse shows. Both were signs to the neurologist that brain repair was happening, something Waller had not dared to anticipate. His educated guess was that other parts of Terry's brain were learning to compensate for what had been destroyed. Waller gives much credit for this to Terry's grim determination to learn to function again.

Waller marvels that Terry got his intelligence back but not his long-term memory. "That's a tough one," he muses, shaking his head. "He's unusual. He's certainly unusual in the amount of recovery he's had. When I first saw him he would stumble over his words. It was hard to follow what he was trying to say. He would use circumlocution – if he couldn't put together the words to say something one way, he'd try another. He was very energetic, so there was a lot of pressure on getting the idea expressed, but he would soon tire and his speech would deteriorate markedly. Now he is articulate and he has a good vocabulary."

He considers. "You have to look at Lorraine for some of the explanation. Most people with brain injuries don't have somebody with Lorraine's patience. She's so important in all this, and he knows that."

Neuroscientists at the Rotman Research Institute in Toronto studied a similar but less devastating case of retrograde amnesia. There, a patient with a damaged right frontal lobe was placed in an MRI tube and given questions requiring verbal responses. The scientists watched something odd – the man's left frontal lobe was lighting up when tasks usually performed by right frontal lobes were called for. The subject's brain was developing new circuitry in the other hemisphere.

Waller likens Terry's development to watching something growing.

"Each time he showed some improvement, and did better than we thought he might, that was encouraging," Waller says. "Every step of the way he kept surprising us at how he was improving. It was a marvellous thing. It really had nothing to do with us, so where did it come from?"

He muses, "There's the drive of nature to fix things up, I suppose, but how does the brain glue itself back together again? We don't know."

Two curious stories of that period concern football. The first involves a "football legends" touch-football game in Hamilton held about two years after Terry's accident. Terry's appearance at the CFL Hall of Fame banquet had lulled the game's sponsors into believing that Terry was restored to his normal self, so he received an invitation to play. He accepted, to Lorraine's alarm, and he asked his oldest daughter Tracy to help him prepare. They found a football and went into the apple orchard to practise. She threw the ball to her father with some of the flare he had taught her. It hit him on the head. Terry had not even put up his hands. Tracy stared aghast at her father, believed by many to be one of the greatest receivers Canadian football has ever known.

"Look, Dad," she said, cupping her hands shoulder high with the wrists apart. "This is how you told me to do it. Let the ball come to you, open your hands, close your fingers, and don't let it go, don't drop it." She threw him a lovely spiral. Although her accuracy was perfect, he missed it again. He had two choices: to quit trying or learn how to do it. For the new Terry as for the old, there was only the latter. Tara and Jennifer were summoned to help, and the three daughters, all of them proficient passers, threw the football to their father for an hour or so. At the end of the practice, he was catching it passably well. And when he turned up in the Hamilton stadium, he put on his football gear, went out on the field with the team and scored the winning touchdown.

"All of a sudden, the ball was there, and my hands were there, and I caught it," he explains, amazed himself. "I made a terrific catch. It just happened, I don't know how."

Some time later J.I. Albrecht phoned him from Sydney, Nova Scotia. Albrecht, a legendary figure in Canadian football history, was aging and had just been hired by a small college in Cape Breton to give them a winning football team. He decided to begin by inviting former football greats to his pre-season camp to show the kids how it was done. Out of affection, he asked Terry Evanshen to coach the young receivers.

Albrecht waited for Terry's plane in the Sydney airport with George Brancato, former Ottawa Rough Rider coach. Lorraine had warned them that Terry would need to be guided or he would lose his way. The two men reflected on the madness of Albrecht's invitation. "Here's a guy who can't find the taxi stand, and we've got him here to teach football," Albrecht groaned.

Their doubts were reinforced when Terry got off the plane wearing a name tag, the kind of identification that airline staff place around the necks of children travelling alone.

The next day on the practice field, however, Terry made a catch on the sidelines that was so brilliant and true that Albrecht gasped. "I swear," he says, "that it was a catch that he might not have made in his playing days." The youngsters on the field stopped in wonder and spontaneously applauded.

For the rest of the day Albrecht watched Terry make all the moves of a fine, thinking receiver. His performance didn't fit with what Albrecht knows about Terry's memory loss. A few times he has tried to talk to Terry about the 1970 Grey Cup–winning Alouette team on which Terry was a receiver and Albrecht the personnel recruiter, but the discussions always are one-sided. "Terry just nods his head and says 'yeah, yeah,'" Albrecht says. "He doesn't remember a thing."

Terry's memory was wiped out, and he travelled with a humiliating name tag around his neck, but he still could play football, a game that requires concentration and planning. How come? Maybe the explanation has to do with patterning. Once Terry is in uniform and running down the field, the pieces of his brain that used to fuse through hundreds of games somehow mesh again to do their old magic. If that is the case, why didn't those pieces co-operate to help him tie his shoes?

Albrecht doesn't want neuroscientists to tell him where certain skills are located in Terry's brain, and which ones can better endure lack of oxygen and a violent shake. The technocrats have nothing to say that Albrecht wants to hear. His explanation for the poetry of Terry's moves on a football field has to do with the glory of the human spirit. He says Terry is just an unusual person. "Football players have to have speed," he explains patiently, "and lots of other measurable factors. Terry had all of them, but then there is the unknown quality, Factor X, which is heart. Terry always had lots of Factor X."

Factor X was getting Terry through frustrations that might have overwhelmed someone with less grit. Once a devoted reader of the *Toronto Star*, the country's largest-circulation newspaper and one with a sizable sports section, Terry found himself unable to follow a story to the second paragraph. "I couldn't get the rhythm of even the first paragraph," he explains. *Rhythm* is a word he uses when he means *sense*. "I couldn't figure out what it was saying. I'd just throw the paper down."

Terry was incapable of divided attention, or making plans, or analysing a situation, or foreseeing consequences, all of which neurologists describe as executive functions. He could learn a task, but three days later he had to learn it again, even though he is an intelligent and adept man. Only with much repetition – twenty to thirty times or more – could his brain move the information or how to perform a simple task into long-term storage so that eventually he do it without supervision.

If distracted in the midst of a chore, he would leave it unfinished and forget that he had started it. The family would find the evidence hours later – a hose running beside the car he had been washing when the phone rang, or doors to the horses' stalls standing open because his attention wandered.

Tracy says of that time, "Before, Dad could do ten things at one time and never be confused. Now he can't watch TV and talk to you at the same time. You can't even ask him a question when he is watching something, because the only answer you'll get – irritably – is 'I'm concentrating.'"

Once when someone wiped mud on the rug by the door, Terry thought Tracy had done it. "He went purple and I could see the pulse pounding in his temples," she says. "He was screaming at me and I was petrified." She started to cry and he ordered her out of the house. He told her to never come back. The next day, when she sat beside him at a friend's wedding, he had forgotten that it had happened.

Eventually the stress was more than Tracy could bear. For a brief period she moved out to work in the kitchen of a nursing home and live with an aunt. But when she developed mononucleosis, it was Terry — somehow rallying his resources beyond anything the family had yet seen — who efficiently made the arrangements to have her admitted to hospital. That's what enabled her to love him again.

When Terry thinks back to that period, he says, "I guess I was a bit nuts. I was really an ugly person. I was angry at myself because I couldn't contribute anything. I was angry that all this crap had made me a lesser person." But he never gave up trying to recover his former skills. Though he had to relearn such mundane tasks as how to make the knot in his tie or write a cheque, he didn't flinch from instruction, and he stayed with each task until he mastered it. And then, since he rarely could repeat the new skill a day later, he would have to be taught the same operation again. And would learn it again. And forget it again. And learn it again.

All this commitment to improving himself was something his family took for granted because Terry had always been like that. Other observers were intrigued that some of the essential Terry Evanshen had made it through the wreckage of his brain. While the destruction of millions of Terry's brain cells had wiped out Terry's gentler qualities and had uncapped unseemly rage, certain fundamentals of his personality had survived. His dominant characteristics from early childhood had been aggressive energy, fearlessness, and stubborn determination to succeed. Possibly he is innately an aggressive man, since some underpinnings of human personality come with the baby, but certainly the competitiveness of his teeming household and impoverished circumstances sharpened whatever infant predilection later drove him to succeed. Terry emerged from his upbringing with a compulsion to excel and an indomitable willingness to do the grunt work that excellence entails. Wherever his instinct to achieve is located in Terry's brain, being blasted out of a Jeep had not touched it at all.

Lorraine noted that as often as he blew up at his family, he was angry at himself more. When Terry was in the fields working alone, she could hear him yelling at the top of his lungs, "Pay attention! *Concentrate!*" If he misplaced something around the house, she could hear him swearing. "I'm such a total loser," he would say aloud. "I'm a loser. I am *stupid*." He says he must have slapped his head ten thousand times in those years.

She tried to comfort him. "You know what," she would begin, as she often does when opening a serious discussion, and taking his hand. "You have this right hand. And every once in a while you have to take it and pat yourself on the shoulder. You have to say to yourself, 'You know what? I'm not such a bad guy.' When you accomplish something, even if you do just a half-assed job, Terry, at this point in time you should pat yourself on the back. Don't be so hard on yourself. We're not all perfect."

He would hang on to her words, silent and sad. "Remember that cake I made yesterday?" she would continue. "I wanted it to rise a whole lot higher, but it didn't. But you know what? It tasted just as good."

Lorraine says, "He was so down on himself, he really couldn't deal with negatives. I tried to keep everything on the positive side." He remembers gratefully how supportive his family was. No matter how much he messed up, Lorraine or one of the daughters would say, "It's all right. Don't think about it. It's all right."

Lorraine observed that Terry was at his worst at the end of the day. Dinner hour, with all three daughters home from school or work, should have been a good time for the family, but instead it was when Terry was most likely to fly into a tantrum. Deciding that he simply was exhausted, Lorraine introduced into his routine an afternoon nap. Terry was hard to convince at first, but he came to love the respite. Every day around four he went to their bedroom and lay down to the soft sounds of relaxation tapes masking noises in the house. Terry rarely slept, but the interlude gave him the immense luxury of not having to concentrate, of letting his mind fall into a restful vacuum. After an hour or two, he would rise refreshed and ready to resume the hard labour of trying to function normally.

Sometimes, when he seemed near the edge of his endurance, Lorraine would coax him to take his nap earlier in the day. If she heard him yelling non-stop at himself, she knew he was reaching the point of collapse. She would hurry to his side. Putting it diplomatically to avoid hurting his feelings, she got him upstairs for a rest.

His only escape from the confusion of his shattered brain was to keep physically busy. In an uncoordinated and often irrational way, he had spurts of cleaning the barn or pruning trees to the nub. Most leisure activities were closed to him. He had no capacity for reflection or daydreaming. He couldn't remember how a book started long enough to make any sense of page five, and he couldn't hold in his head the early scenes of a new movie in order to understand ten minutes later what all those people were doing. Empty-content, facile television worked better, and he became addicted to the news. What also worked well was the repetition of favourite films he could watch in the family's den.

Terry has seen Robert De Niro in *Midnight Run* maybe two hundred times. Nights when he couldn't sleep and had finished his walk, he would load the VCR with *Midnight Run*, and sit back contentedly. He can never tire of it because much of the story comes up fresh and new for him every time. The rest of the Evanshens grew so sick of *Midnight Run* that no one would stay in the same room when the tape was playing, but he was insatiable.

In the dark hours before dawn, Lorraine would often find him downstairs watching *Midnight Run*, and would urge him to return to bed. He would brush her off. He couldn't leave before the film's end, his favourite part, the one bit he has memorized. "It's about friendship," he explains earnestly. "I have to see the end, where he gives him the money, and then he disappears. And De Niro walks out and he hails a cab. And he says to the guy, 'Have you got change for a thousand dollars?' And the guy says, 'Are you crazy!' And De Niro says, 'Get outta here. I'm walkin'.' And he starts walking down the road."

Terry's face glows when he describes the movie's ending; something about it strikes a deep chord. Why does he like it so much? "Well," he begins awkwardly, "there's friendship." He searches for the words he wants. "And there's the sense of purpose about what he wanted to do. And he *did* it. He's walking with strength . . ." Terry gives up, but he is beaming. "I don't know why, I just really enjoy it."

He enjoys it because it's really about his dream for himself. It's about a man who overcomes adversity and at the end of his ordeal he saunters down the road, intact and independent.

Sometimes, loving that part so much, Terry would brush off Lorraine's sleepy objections and start the film again from the beginning. To watch over him and keep him safe, Lorraine would make herself a cup of tea, stretch out on the couch in the living room, leaving open the doors between them, and drink her tea and doze until he was ready to go back to bed.

Gradually Terry accumulated a number of other videos, choosing films he had enjoyed on those nights when the family went to the movies. He couldn't follow the plot in the movie theatre and didn't try, knowing the effort to be hopeless, but he always was left with an impression of whether it was a good film or one that he didn't like. He wrote down the titles of those he remembered enjoying, and would wait for those films to turn up at his neighbourhood video outlet. Loading the tape in his VCR, he would watch the new film twenty times, gradually getting some sense of what it was about. If the film starred Robert De Niro, a tough, indomitable small man with whom Terry identifies intensely, he'd play it fifty times.

To combat the panic and embarrassment he felt when meeting people who knew him before the accident and wanted to talk about old times, Terry was struggling to memorize stories about himself that he could tell in social encounters. He watched videos of himself playing football, and he admired the man who was said to be him. Sometimes he felt a kinetic connection, and would twist his body the way the man did to avoid a tackle. Over and over, the family showed him photo albums, scrapbooks, and tapes of such events as his wedding and birthday parties. The man in the photos and on the screen looked like him: in fact, he certainly was him because Terry saw the same face in his shaving mirror. But nothing was familiar, including the person who clearly was himself. He searched earnestly to find something, perhaps in the background, that might trigger a flash of recall, but his efforts were hopeless. His previous existence simply was not accessible to him, however vivid the evidence. Terry might as well have been leafing through the family albums of a boring stranger.

Medical archives contain a case with strong resemblances to Terry's situation. J.V., a fifty-year-old man who suffered multiple seizures and lost all his memories prior to 1982, was studied at length by Rotman Institute neuropsychologist Donald Stuss and neurologist Antonio Guzman of the University of Ottawa. Unlike Terry, J.V.'s capacity to store and retrieve new memories worked at near normal levels once the seizures were controlled, but family albums meant as little to him as they did to Terry. The two scientists noted, in the journal *Brain and Cognition*, that J.V. had no feeling of warmth about the things he learned about himself from his family or from looking at photographs. As for recalling incidents of his past service in the navy, that was out of the question. He didn't even remember being in the navy.

The stories about himself that Terry enjoyed most concerned football. Family members tried to teach him about his childhood and the good times in the years since his marriage, but those tales didn't touch him and were harder to hold in his new memory than the football anecdotes. Even so, the football stories that he has learned to repeat have an eerie flatness. Terry can't fill in what others have failed to mention, as people with normal memories do when someone prompts them to recall an event such as a canoe trip. A reference to, say, "that weekend at Big Trout Lake" brings the forest into the mind's eye of everyone who was there — the night it rained, the sound of cold water trickling over stones, the moose standing in the shallows. The stories Terry hears about himself have no such dimension. They never awakened the event for him. He can't visualize the setting, or hear the laughter, or see the faces. Informed about a touchdown he made in a difficult circumstance, he can memorize the fact that he did it, but he doesn't hear the crowd cheer.

"I had a lot of great people live those football memories with me," he explains. "They tell me stories. I can't add anything to the story because I'm not there. I can only laugh at it."

This would make perfect sense to the neuropsychologist Dr. Brian Levine and his associates at the Rotman Research Institute. Levine had a case much like Terry's and found in the literature a number of similar cases dating back to 1982. He comments, "Even when patients learn and retain information about personal past events, they consistently report an inability to re-experience these events as part of their own subjective past; the events may just as well have happened to someone else."

In time Terry accrued a repertoire of stories about himself that he could recite at appropriate moments. When interviewed by the media or in a conversation about sport, he could say with confidence that he fumbled the ball only three times in his four-teen-year career, or that he once scored four touchdowns in a single game, or that he talked J.I. Albrecht into giving him a tryout in Montreal when he was only an eighteen-year-old lightweight.

If pressed for details about these events, he rarely admitted that he really didn't remember the episode at all, or that he was only reciting what he had been told by people he trusted to give him a true account. Most often his reaction to a request to elaborate was to behave as if he hadn't heard the question. He would tell another memorized story and ease away. During several television interviews he did in that period, Terry forgot the question before he opened his mouth to answer. With a trapped expression in his eyes, he would tell an irrelevant football story while the interviewer's face registered bewilderment.

People who spent any amount of time with Terry came to see that his anecdotes were only practised words he strung together. The tipoff was, and still is, that he told each story exactly the same way every time, word for word. His family, friends, and therapists could recite a dozen of his stories right along with him if they chose to do so. Like an actor delivering lines, Terry is a prisoner of a script someone has handed him, which he can't embellish or edit. One friend timed his delivery, and marvelled at the consistency: a story took exactly the same number of minutes in every telling.

If interrupted in the recounting of his set pieces, Terry is obliged to start again from the beginning. The distraction shatters his concentration and he is unable to pick up from where the interjection occurred. Requests to elaborate on an incident – *Who was the coach then?* – upset him. He doesn't know.

The emptiness in which Terry dwells is not total. Sometimes ghosts walk. Once something popped into his head for no reason he could see. Suddenly he got a sense of himself in football uniform out on an open field on a wintry day, with the cold so intense he was in pain. He couldn't picture the setting – not the stadium or even which team uniform he was wearing – but he suddenly knew the misery of a time in his past when his feet and bare hands were beginning to freeze. Maybe it was the game in Regina when he broke his leg. Someone once told him it was cruelly cold that day. Maybe it was during one of the two Grey

Cup finals he played. He can't fill in the picture. But the memory of being cold was real, and for one exquisite moment he was united with his former self. He can't summon that moment back, but he will never forget that it happened.

Every month or so for years after the accident, Terry got another kind of reminder. He would feel a twinge in his left arm and find that another piece of glass was working itself through the skin. An orthopaedic surgeon estimated that Terry had almost a hundred bits of glass in that arm, and his left elbow was constantly sore. Routinely, Terry popped into a hospital emergency department to have glass removed or the possible tendinitis explored.

The Evanshens' money difficulties were mounting again, with no sign that the insurance companies were ready to concede that the Evanshens deserved anything near the $2 million that Bernie Gluckstein was asking. By means of threats that damages would pile up, the lawyer sometimes obtained an advance payment, but these concessions were always insufficient to meet the Evanshens' debt. Lorraine was impatient with the slowness of the process but Gluckstein explained that waiting for court days on a crowded docket was something that happened to everyone, and further delays were being caused by the obstructionist tactics of the insurance companies.

Many people involved in claims for long-term disability have horror stories to tell of the stalling and mean-minded practices of insurance companies across Canada, especially when personal injuries are involved, and there is an increasing clamour that the industry be investigated. In most provinces, the laws seem to favour insurance companies over injured people. Ontario's "no-fault" plan for automobile accidents, established two years after Terry's accident, cut deeply into litigation costs, but two revisions to that legislation since have created bewildering paperwork for everyone and have made life infinitely more beautiful for insurance companies.

Gluckstein could write a textbook on the subject. In fact, he has written numerous articles in legal and neurological journals on the topics of dealing with insurance companies and representing brain-injured clients. He is frank about the challenges. In a 1995 issue of the Houston-based *i.e. Magazine* he wrote, "Their [brain-injured clients'] volatility and rigidity make them very difficult to deal with. Their problems with memory and concentration sometimes make them unreliable and their problems with execution make it very difficult for them to follow through on legal advice and direction."

His problems with Terry were minor in comparison. With him, Terry was an agreeable and submissive man. It was Lorraine who was doing the fuming. The annual cost of running the farm alone was around $35,000 – and there were the family's living expenses on top of that. Terry was receiving a modest disability payment from his government pension fund, but this did not begin to cover their costs, and his Canadian Football League pension would not kick in until he was fifty-five years old. Lorraine was mortified and frightened that at times her line of credit at the bank rose astronomically. She wanted resolution of the case but all that was happening, so far as she could see, was a series of affidavits and discovery hearings – and a lot of meetings.

The bulk of the compensation Gluckstein was seeking would be based on a calculation of Terry's loss of income since the accident and an estimate of his future earnings had he not been injured. That meant that Terry would have to be convincing in court as a profoundly disabled man, something he never appears to be on first sight. Gluckstein, however, had decided that if the case went to trial, Terry would be his first witness. The lawyer had no concern that Terry could seem too poised and collected to be believable as a man who could never again be employed. All that had to happen, Gluckstein knew, was for the insurance company lawyers to keep Terry on the stand a long time, as he expected they would. Terry most certainly would tire, lose his concentration, and either blow up or ramble.

During Terry's appearance at a discovery hearing, this was exactly what happened. Gluckstein warned the opposing lawyers not to push Terry around with belligerent questions, but they ignored his caution. During a protracted line of questioning about his former employment, Terry offered to punch the insurance company lawyer in the nose. Gluckstein walked him out.

While accountants hired by Gluckstein were putting together estimates of what Terry's earnings might have been if the accident had not happened, something fortuitous occurred. Terry was approached by a headhunter, Robert Short, a former vice-president of CNCP Telecommunications when Terry worked there. Aware of Terry's accident but not of the consequences, Short wanted to know if Terry was available to apply for a job as the Canadian general manager for a U.S. company involved in data transmission. His base annual salary would be $90,000, with the expectation that commissions and other benefits would make the total close to $125,000 a year.

Terry, frightened but hopeful, asked Barbara Baptiste to go with him to see Short. The interview was a disaster. Short commented afterwards, "It was sad to note that clearly his physical condition would not now permit him to take on the responsibility of this type of position." Nevertheless, Short had given the Evanshens – and their lawyer – a benchmark to compute his lost salary potential.

The constant concern about money was fraying Lorraine's nerves, exacerbating the manifest difficulty of living with Terry. More than two years had passed since the accident, and the family of five was still living without sufficient income. At one point, the debt climbed into six figures and the bank indicated reluctance to continue the line of credit. Lorraine noticed her daughters withdrawing into themselves, and saw herself becoming bad-tempered. Something had to change, but Barbara Baptiste had canvassed the whole country without finding any rehabilitation program that would do more for Terry than therapies she had been able to cobble together in Toronto.

Towards the end of 1990, two and a half years after Terry's accident, Lorraine realized she was too worn out to continue much longer as Terry's principal therapist and caregiver. For a while there was talk of hiring a companion, but that plan fell through for lack of money. As far as Lorraine could see, Terry's condition was almost unchanged. He had acquired some practised civilities, to be sure, and he had a fine repertoire of football stories, but he still slept only in two-hour stretches, his embraces were artificial, and their resumed sexual relationship was a rare, cold, utilitarian union totally unlike the sensitive love-making she had known. Most distressing of all, his temper was still on a hair-trigger and she couldn't remember when she ever had been relaxed in his company.

She pleaded with Barbara Baptiste to find help – anywhere. Baptiste had just heard of a brain-injury rehabilitation program, the

Casa Colina Transitional Living Center in Pomona, California. She arranged for Dr. Roger Wood, a neuropsychologist and the clinical director of the centre, to examine Terry and review his medical and psychological profile with a view to having him admitted. Wood did so in May 1990, and delivered a diagnosis that was precise on some points and vague on others.

He observed in Terry a "general pattern orbito-frontal injury complicated either by cerebral hypoxia or diffuse axonal injury, or both" – and turned him down. The California program would not be able to benefit someone as damaged as Terry, he said. However, Wood recommended that Baptiste try someone just up the coast, Dr. Catherine Mateer, known to everyone as Katy, who was said to be one of about ten top clinical neuropsychologists in the world. She later moved to Canada and took up the position of professor and director of clinical training at the University of Victoria, but at the time she was in Washington State, running a comprehensive residential treatment program for brain-damaged people. Bernie Gluckstein, who has some authority in this field, describes Mateer at that time as "the best cognitive therapist in North America."

Mateer, who once suffered a brain injury herself, worked at the Good Samaritan Hospital Center for Cognitive Rehabilitation in Puyallup, on the outskirts of Seattle, Washington, where she headed a holistic program that offered cognitive therapy five days a week, with six therapists a day, each session lasting one hour. It addressed psychosocial problems, verbal fluency, memory stretching, vocational and recreational needs, and helped with practical matters such as money and household management, parenting, meal preparation, and shopping.

"Good Sam," as Lorraine calls it, requires its clients to live for six to eight months independently of their families in small apartments under the eye of a resident supervisor, where they must demonstrate an ability to look after themselves. It sounded impressive but first there had to be screening to determine if Terry was a suitable candidate.

In Terry's file the evaluation team from Good Sam found as dismal a medical history as it had ever seen. In brusque language, a summary of Terry's many difficulties stated in part:

"At the present time, physical problems are reported to include insomnia, restlessness, back and neck pain, reduced flexibility, decreased coordination and speed of performance, impaired balance, and blurred vision. Identified cognitive deficits include problems with concentration and attention, memory problems, retrograde amnesia, mild word-finding problems, slowed speed of performance, and periods of confusion. Also reported are psychosocial problems characterized by increased irritability, reduced tolerance for frustration, a quickness to anger, compulsive orderliness, social withdrawal, and depression."

Terry saw the Good Samaritan Hospital as his only hope, and was ready to give the assessment his best. Mateer, who conducted the evaluation with a team of colleagues, noted that he was "open and co-operative" and "a personable, socially adept man." They attributed this poise to his years of being in the public eye. Only after talking with him for a while did the image of a capable, confident man fall apart. They were touched to see tears in his eyes when an assigned task proved too difficult.

The assessment included a stream of interviews and fifteen tests, some of them repeated a few times and one of them taking three hours. Terry's performance in such areas as memory, intelligence, and new learning skills measured in the low range, the intelligence score lower than had been tested elsewhere, possibly from nervousness or fatigue. The phrase "severely impaired" appears frequently in the summary of his test results. Katy Mateer also discovered something not included routinely in Terry's documents: his "substantial" loss of biographical memory – marriage, football, schools, his father's death, his children's birth, employment, all gone. "This is obviously greatly disturbing to him," Mateer wrote sympathetically. "It [the amnesia] will likely be permanent."

Terry proved to be aware that his family relationships were teetering. Admitting candidly that he was in trouble with his wife and children, he blamed only himself. He said he was far too critical – "nit-picking" – and worried that his family was "tired" of him. Mostly he was disturbed that he often fought with his wife, something he had been told rarely happened before the accident.

In the end, Mateer and her colleagues decided the brain injury day-treatment program at the Good Samaritan Hospital might help Terry, and his name was placed on a waiting list.

The hitch was that the Good Samaritan's program would cost approximately forty thousand dollars in U.S. funds over the six-month period, plus travel and living expenses, and the expense would not be covered by the public Ontario Health Insurance Plan because the treatment centre was in the United States. Exceptions have been made, however, for out-of-country care when appropriate and vitally needed treatment is not available in Canada. The Evanshens would have to convince OHIP that Terry's only hope for rehabilitation was in the States.

After much pressure from Barbara Baptiste, an OHIP panel convened for a special hearing, an unusual accommodation in itself. Baptiste testified that Terry had been using all the applicable treatment services in the Toronto and Oshawa area for more than two years with little improvement, and Ray Remple, then executive director of the Ontario Head Injury Association, told the tribunal that there was nothing to help Terry anywhere else in Canada either.

Baptiste says that Remple was "a phenomenal advocate," adding, "Just even having him there was a big help, but also he spoke so well." The two authorities on brain injury told the tribunal that Terry had improved a lot, thanks to his own grim perseverance, his supportive family, and the best therapy that could be found, but still his frustration was mounting because of the limited number of things he could do. Tactfully, they let the tribunal know that Lorraine was nearly at the end of her rope.

One of people on the OHIP panel made a dismissive comment about Baptiste "demanding" a service. She cut in. "We're not demanding. Please understand that we're not demanding," she said levelly. "This is a *request.*"

She explained that Terry's brain injury was unusual because it was a combination of three factors, each of them appalling in itself. Along with the contusion in the frontal lobe area and the oxygen deprivation, he had suffered diffuse axonal injury. "With all the straining and shearing that happened to the bundles of neurons in his brain when he was thrown through the Jeep," she explained, "the injury became diffuse. It's not like you've had a stroke or something where it's quite focal. What happens to your head in a car accident when vehicles are moving at speed is like falling eight storeys."

Her testimony was reinforced by a stack of documentation about Terry's condition signed by his medical doctors and other therapists. The letter from Doug Waller was particularly eloquent. He wrote: "Mr. Evanshen is a national hero. . . . Ms. Baptiste has struggled relentlessly to find every possible method of treatment that could be used to help Mr. Evanshen. . . . He still is, as he was, an exceptional Canadian and I think he deserves to be given every opportunity we can find for him."

In the face of such overwhelming evidence, OHIP agreed to pay for Terry's treatment at Good Sam. After four months on the waiting list, Terry was notified that an opening was available. Barbara Baptiste made the arrangements for Terry's Canada Pension Plan disability cheques to be deposited in a bank in Puyallup, obtained the proper documents for the U.S. Immigration officials at the border, and made contact with an American family physician who would monitor Terry's physical condition while he was away.

Lorraine's mood swung between elation and panic. Good Sam would mean a six-month reprieve from the strain of living with Terry, but also six months of fretting. Terry never cooked for himself, for instance; if she didn't prepare a meal for him he didn't eat at all. He said he found it too difficult to follow a recipe or remember what ingredients were already in the mix. Lorraine had a not-unreasonable fear that he might get absent-minded around the stove and either burn himself or set fire to the apartment. And how would be find his way alone in a strange city? Across a bridge that might lure him to jump?

Despite her worries, Lorraine and their daughters saw Terry off on February 19, 1991, at Toronto's Pearson International Airport. They were full of anxiety and tenderness when they watched him leave, but the emotion that won out when they returned to an empty house was jubilation. That evening Lorraine and her daughters ate a leisurely late dinner, put on their night clothes and romped around the living room like kids let out of school.

The objectives established at the Good Samaritan Hospital's Center for Cognitive Rehabilitation for Terry included improvement to his attention span and concentration, and teaching him to compensate for his short-term memory problems. A heavy emphasis was placed on making him fit to return to work and helping him have a better relationship with his family. The techniques incorporated simulated workplace and social situations, individual therapy sessions, and group therapy.

Group therapy appalled Terry. "All these people sitting around complaining, telling their troubles," he says indignantly. "I wasn't going to do that!"

He was told he had to do it, and it was explained to him that others in the group were not complaining, they simply were revealing their true feelings. Terry was profoundly disgusted at the suggestion that he should reveal his true feelings, especially to strangers. He had never been a complainer, he said angrily, and he wasn't going to start. Offended one day by a doleful recital in the group, Terry yelled at the hapless man, "*I'm tired of all your bullshit! You've got no problems compared to my problems.*"

Mateer prudently decided Terry was unsuited to group therapy. She abandoned the effort and increased the number of his one-on-one sessions instead.

The spartan apartment Terry rented was inspected weekly by someone from the CCR to see if he was learning to care for himself. He certainly was. Keeping it immaculate was not a problem, since he could tolerate nothing less, and he had solved the problem of cooking by eating inexpensive meals every day at a nearby Chinese restaurant where the husband-wife proprietors understood his condition and were kind. He walked to the hospital for his daily regimen with a map in his hand.

Lorraine phoned him three evenings a week. The conversations were brief because Terry always sounded exhausted. Karyn Ottolino, an occupational therapist and program manager assigned to Terry, observed that he was working very hard in order to appear normal, and this was "very fatiguing and frustrating for him." She added, "He has noted to us that he tends to withdraw and socially isolate himself because of the stress this places on him."

But Terry was enthusiastic about the possibility that he would improve greatly at Good Sam. He wanted Lorraine and the girls to move to Vancouver so he could be closer to the hospital, and he announced he might even find employment with his brother Frank. Lorraine without hesitation put the farm up for sale, though the country's economy was in a slump and the real estate market was dismal.

Five months into the program, Terry changed his mind about his prospects. He could see that it was unrealistic to expect that he could work for his brother, although he had made some improvements in his independence. He had picked up some tips about using a Daytimer to help him keep on track. He had been advised to purchase a filing cabinet and taught to store information by categories in it, and he had developed some skills at refinishing antiques during a vocational and recreational rehabilitation program. His attention span had improved slightly and he was learning the trick of calming himself by double exhaling when frustrated. He truly enjoyed a volunteer "work station" placement at a fitness club, which was designed to test his work habits and ability to control his temper. Terry was found to be incapable of tasks such as taking telephone calls or scheduling appointments, which require compartmented thinking, but he could manage simple responsibilities. His hours at the club were increased gradually, and his limit was found to be a five-hour day two days running, and no more. After that he was either too depleted to function or he blew up over trivialities.

Although five hours of "being nice" represented a victory of sorts, Terry was discouraged. The effort to meet his own expectations was too draining and he felt himself close to cracking. In some ways, he believed himself to be regressing and he was ready to quit. He told Lorraine to take down the For Sale sign on the farm. He was coming home.

Noting his despondent state of mind, Katy Mateer had a talk with him and spotted the problem. Terry wasn't homesick for his family so much as he was lonely for himself. He missed the person he had been before the accident and he was losing hope that he would ever become that person again. She gave him some thoughtful advice. "I can tell you what's wrong with you medically," she said, "but personally I believe character is not a piece of your brain or a part of your heart. Maybe it's the soul that people talk about. Character lasts. Don't question it. Your character from before is going to start coming back through again."

Terry didn't believe her. It had been three years since the accident and he could see little sign of any former character coming through, unless his former self was a miserable, explosive jerk.

The next morning, a Saturday, he refused to join a group outing to a movie and instead sat by himself watching a sports show on television. The great pitcher Nolan Ryan was being interviewed following his seventh no-hitter. He was asked, "Nolan, how do you approach baseball?" Ryan took a baseball, assumed a pitcher's stance and started his windup. Then he said, as Terry remembers it, "This pitch, this moment, is my total commitment to every single windup. I try to put everything I have into each and every pitch that I throw. I have only one gear. If I have control of my windup, I do not fear the opposition."

Terry sat bolt upright. *That's me!* he thought. "That's how I played football. I was focussed and I did not fear anyone."

This moment of recognizing himself in Nolan Ryan was the turning point for Terry, as he says repeatedly. A sense of vast relief drenched him in joy. He felt connected to his former self, and that epiphany marked the beginning of an ambition to become a second Terry Evanshen who would be as worthy of esteem as the first. He says that's when he realized he needed to give up wanting to be the first Terry Evanshen, but he could aspire to being just as commendable – only different. He decided, as he puts it every time he tells this story, "to take one day at a time and rebuild the new Terry, because I can't touch the guy from yesterday."

Katy Mateer had been trying to tell him that. "It's like being an alcoholic," she told him. "You have to accept the facts and start going forward." Now he knew what she meant. He said to himself, "Jeez, Terry, you can do that. You better start listening to what they've been trying to teach you for the last five months. Take one day at a time and rebuild the new Terry because you can't touch the guy from yesterday."

When Nolan Ryan heard of his effect on Terry, he sent him an autographed baseball.

Though Terry counts that moment as turning his life around, he owes his present state equally to something else that happened at Good Sam – a visit from a former Alouette teammate, Ron

Perowne. Perowne, his wife, Gail, and their three children, aged fifteen, thirteen, and six, were driving home from a visit to some relatives in Portland, Oregon, and happened to pass through Puyallup. Perowne, a wide receiver of about Terry's size, with sandy, tousled hair and a friendly, muddled face that has earned him the nickname Popeye, made the Alouettes in 1972 through a series of flukes — a trade here, an injury there — that left the team desperate for a receiver. Perowne still maintains modestly that he could never have made the team under normal circumstances. He went to his first practice with the nervous conviction he was out of his league. Terry Evanshen, whom Perowne idolized, was the first to shake his hand and introduce himself.

"Welcome," Terry said warmly. "If you have any questions, you come to me. If I have any observations, I'll come to you."

That considerate gesture stayed with Perowne long after he left football. When he read of Terry's accident, he phoned Lorraine to commiserate and he kept in touch afterwards. He knew Terry was at the Good Samaritan hospital and he insisted that his family should stop and have dinner with him. His children groaned. Dinner with a strange adult was not high on their list of vacation treats. Perowne made the call anyway and the two men agreed on a restaurant where they all would meet.

Perowne's encounter with Terry happened soon after his click of self-recognition during the Nolan Ryan interview. Terry was on a high. Gone was the morose, resentful Evanshen, and on deck was a relentlessly cheerful, optimistic man. He was bearing down in the therapy sessions, eagerly lapping up whatever Good Sam had to teach him. He was enthusiastically studying written suggestions for ways to handle social situations. If asked about his brain damage, he had learned that he didn't have to discuss it. He could deflect the question with, "I'm doing fine now, and how are things with you and your family?" People who asked what was wrong with his memory could be put off with, "Recovery is a life-long process," or "I can't explain it. Some things are still not known." If Terry was giving a speech or interview, something not outside the realm of possibility for a man who still had a public profile in Canada, therapists told him to frame his brain injury as a challenge he was fighting to overcome.

He had a printed sheet with all these suggestions, which he rehearsed frequently in the hope of memorizing them. The last advice suited him perfectly. Fighting challenges had been his specialty since he learned to walk.

Terry sailed into dinner with the Perowne family at the top of his form. He was expansive, he was charming, and he talked at length about the challenges of being brain-injured and his fight to overcome them. The Perownes were enthralled – especially, as Ron and Gail could not help but note, their three children. Two and a half hours flew by with the youngsters, normally restless in the presence of a talkative adult, a rapt audience. When the family continued on its way it was obvious that the children were very moved.

It gave Ron Perowne an idea. He once studied theology and he is an idealist, always on the lookout for stories of heroic endeavour that lift the human spirit. What Terry Evanshen should do with his second life, he decided, was give speeches to young people and inspire them to try harder. And he knew exactly where Terry could begin.

NINE

On August 15, 1991, Terry returned from the Good Samaritan program to a well-rested family. They were happy to have him home but also apprehensive that they would be plunged again into the wariness and fatigue of living with an unpredictable man. After a week or so Lorraine and the daughters privately concluded that the improvements he had made were certainly noticeable but were not hugely significant.

On the good side, Terry seemed more controlled than he had been and more focussed. He was using a notebook to steer him through daily tasks and he referred constantly to his Daytimer. That was some progress, and he was showing a degree of interest in his daughters' activities, which was also was new. Another notable change was that he was speaking more slowly, which meant that he was more coherent and slurred his words less. But they had hoped for so much more, even imagining that he might be his old self again – affectionate, spontaneous, capable. Instead he was still bad-tempered, obsessive, and preoccupied with himself. They did not discuss their disappointment, but quietly went back to the hard work of trying to keep him calm.

Terry didn't notice their gloom. For the most part, he was in a state of euphoric optimism, and declared that this was only the beginning of his recovery. That mood lasted only a short time. Almost overnight Terry's ebullience waned, and then vanished. Back in his home setting, he could see that what he had acquired at Good Sam was not much more than a collection of tricks. He understood suddenly that he would never have the competence he had been dreaming about. He would never recover enough to hold a job again or be an independent man. The realization plunged him into despair.

Many neuropsychologists doubt that neuroclinics such as the one at Good Sam have much to offer to people with broken brains. The ability to heal a brain really is not within the staff's expertise, or anyone's. What they do, and often quite effectively, is help brain-damaged people compensate and adjust to living with their disabilities. By means of repetitive exercises and such aids as daily journals, people gain a small, consoling sense of control over the chaos in their heads, but the profound neural disruption that causes their difficulties in the first place is not much altered in therapy.

Neuropsychologists McKay Moore Sohlberg and Catherine Mateer, both of them at Good Samaritan Hospital, and Donald Stuss of the Rotman Research Institute, report in the paper "Introduction to Cognitive Rehabilitation" that head-trauma treatment programs are aimed in good part at making brain-damaged people easier to be around. They teach injured people to be more respectful of others and to express themselves more clearly. Among the strategies therapists advise are the use of wall charts, memory boards, calendars, reminders to take the house key tacked to the inside of the front door, photographs of friends with their names taped on, and regular routines. Families are warned that brain-damaged people are easily upset by the unexpected and there isn't much point in telling the injured person that the week after next is Mother's birthday, because "the week after next" is a meaningless concept.

Follow-up studies of the lasting effects of cognitive treatment are in their infancy and there is little assurance that the modifications are permanent. In any case, improvements in the unhappy subjects are rarely dramatic and seem as much influenced by health, age, lifestyle, and family support as by anything the diligent therapists can do. Nonetheless, even small gains means a great deal to reduce a subject's depression and enable relatives to keep hope alive.

In their paper, Sohlberg, Mateer, and Stuss state, "Although impairments in such functions as anticipation, goal selection, planning, self-regulation, incorporating feed-back, and completion of intended activities are prevalent following head injury [to the frontal lobes], remediation efforts have been fairly minimal."

Terry's expectations of what Good Sam could do had been overly optimistic and the return to the reality of his limited existence was more than he could bear. He was overwhelmed by hopelessness. "He seemed to understand the extent of his injuries for the first time," Lorraine comments. "He came to accept the deficits that would always be there."

Terry says of this period, "Everything was crap again. There was nothing good in my life, no balance. I wasn't doing anything right. And how would I ever do anything right when I didn't understand anything?" He saw himself as a man without a single redeeming feature. He knew he once had been a loving, happy person, and he yearned for that man as people do for a lost love, but the new Evanshen was a sour, unpleasant person. "I banged my head ten thousand times," he said. "Saying *you stupid dummy.*"

Something drove him to keep trying, and his family got behind that compulsion. His daughters fed back to him the lines he used when they were competing in sports: "You've got to do your best," they said to him. "Never give up. Come on, Dad. You always told us we should never give up, so you have to keep going."

They were growing up and appreciating better that Lorraine needed their help. Their greatest fear, which they shared with one another, was that she would collapse and leave the care of their father entirely to them. Lorraine's exhaustion and growing testiness frightened them, but she rarely admitted she was near the end of her rope. Only occasionally would she say, "I'm really whipped today, girls. You're going to have to spend a little time with Dad. Maybe go for a walk with him, give him a pep talk. Because I'm finished."

No one in the Evanshen family is a quitter, but the gloomy, withdrawn expression on Terry's face began to depress them all. One Sunday afternoon Lorraine found him in the kitchen with a list of small tasks in his hand, checking off what he had done and reviewing what remained. He looked up at her with empty eyes. Impulsively, she sat beside him and said, "Don't interrupt me. I have something to say and it might take a while.

"Y'know Terry, this has been one hell of a blow for all of us. There's no doubt about it. But you know what? The world doesn't stop because you have had an accident. We have to go on, and in order for us to do that we need for you to get up off your butt. You used to be a man with a big smile on your face. Now we never see you smile, and when you go around scowling you make the rest of us feel bad too. When you're down, everybody gets down. Please search every day for a happy thought and put that smile back on your face."

Terry smiled at her, a not bad effort, and went quietly upstairs to think about what she had said. He looked at himself in the mirror and decided, as he tells it, that he had been selfish. Everyone was helping him, but he wasn't helping anyone. "The girls had been getting up at five-thirty to feed the horses before coming back to shower and eat and go off to school. I realized I'd been stealing time from them. Everyone was trying to help me and I was nothing but a pain in the neck."

Around four the next morning, unable to sleep, he crept out of bed, found his clothes, wrote a note he left on the kitchen table, and went out to the barn to clean the stalls and feed the horses.

When they came down for breakfast the family was electrified. Terry was gone and the note said that his daughters could go back to bed. When he returned to the house he announced he would be mucking out the stalls from then on, and he would feed the dogs (Tara estimates there were eleven at that time) and the cats (including a new litter), and he would be mowing the lawn and repairing the wooden fences, and he would prune the twenty-three apple trees. To demonstrate his new helpfulness, he jumped up from the massive oak kitchen table where the family was eating and began washing the dishes before the others had even finished their meal.

His lassitude was gone. Now he was a dervish, seized with ferocious energy and particular about his appearance to a fault. Lorraine says, "His grooming became almost obsessive – the cleaning of the toenails, the fingernails, the cream on his face . . ." She groans. His perfectionism made every task take a very long time. Where before the accident he had mowed the huge lawn in two hours, he now took two days. He pruned the apple trees almost to their roots, taking a long time to do it. He was never still.

The key to the overnight change might well have been Lorraine's astute comment that once he had been a smiling man. Nothing commands Terry's attention more than information about the man he was before the accident, and little in his life means more to him than imitating that man's behaviour as best he can. If he used to have a smile on his face, he would put a smile on his face; if he used to pull his weight with chores, he would do the chores.

In a moment of poignant candour, he once said, "Every day, I'm an actor. They give me a script and I read the script, but I can't be the director and disagree."

Days when he could find nothing at the farm that urgently needed to be fixed, rearranged or pruned, he would drive to downtown Toronto by quiet back roads, a route he had travelled so many times he could do it without getting lost. He parked in the same lot he always used, where the attendant knew that sometimes he could not find his car, and then he would sit with a cup of coffee in a café opposite his lawyer's office, the one place in Toronto he could find easily, simply watching the life on the street. After a while, he would drive home. It was something to do, and it gave him a sense of control.

The bursts of activity around the farm may have been more than his damaged frame could bear. Lorraine noted that he seemed to be in physical agony. Terry's pain threshold is unusually high. He's a stoic who won't readily confess when he is hurting, but Lorraine could see him wince whenever he stood up or bent over. Finally he acknowledged that his back and neck were making him miserable.

Lorraine told Barbara Baptiste, who recommended Dr. Gary
Adams, a chiropractor in Whitby who was making a specialty of
treating people who had been involved in car accidents, and also
was branching into rehabilitation. Adams, then in his early
forties, is a charming and perceptive man with a well-trimmed
dark beard and an easy manner. He first saw Terry in September
1991 and decided that the injuries Terry's spine sustained in the
accident were just short of a fracture. The compression and
torque from the collision, combined with the battering to his
neck and back from football, had severely punished his spinal
column. The fact that his spine didn't break in the accident
probably owes something to his unusual muscular development.
Adams thinks that Terry came as close to being paralysed as a
person can be and still walk. While the chiropractor found
Terry's mobility a miracle in itself, he also marvelled that a man
with such an acutely damaged brain would seem at first glance
to be a normal person

"I really didn't have a clue about how much I could help
him," Adams confesses. "I hoped that I could give him a bit of
relief from the discomfort he was experiencing, but I was hesitant
about what I could really accomplish. And he seemed in such a
sad state when he came in. He had a map of how to get to my
office in his hand, and directions on how to get home. He was
very withdrawn, and he didn't have many social graces."

After a few months of regular adjustments, with Adams
working to unlock Terry's neck and his spine's poor alignment,
Terry reported that he felt better, had more energy, and was sleeping for longer periods – sometimes for as much as three hours at a
stretch. Adams was greatly encouraged, and so was Barbara
Baptiste, who was monitoring Terry's treatment.

One day Baptiste surprised Adams by asking if Terry could work in the clinic as a volunteer. Terry needed some training in social interaction to help him regain his civility, she explained, and Lorraine desperately needed time to herself. Baptiste picked Adams because Terry liked and trusted the chiropractor and would therefore be comfortable in his office, and because she knew intuitively that Adams was the kind of person who would say yes. Adams agreed, not without trepidation, to use Terry on a trial basis as the office greeter.

"Terry was even then a very likeable individual," Adams says, explaining why he took the chance, "but he was like a cat in a cage. He needed an outlet, and it was his sincerity that made me want to work with him. He was really trying. But, to be honest, I had no idea how it would turn out."

Twice a week Terry went to the clinic for an hour or so. His role was to summon patients whose turn came for treatments. He would go into the waiting room and ask newcomers their name. Then he would say, "Hello, I'm happy to meet you. My name is Terry Evanshen. I'm helping out here. Dr. Adams is ready. Would you come with me?" He wrote every word on a card, including "My name is Terry Evanshen," and read it stiffly. Between patients, he sat by himself and studied the card.

"Believe me," he said later, "just introducing myself and asking for names was a huge accomplishment."

Bernie Gluckstein had delegated his lawyer-associate, Fern Silverman, to prepare accounting-firm documents and employer affidavits. The estimate of Terry's loss of income in the three years since the accident was $225,000, and by the same calculations, if he was unable to be employed again, his loss of future income until retirement age was set at $1,241,244. The insurance companies were appalled. His placement as a volunteer receptionist led them to wonder whether Terry might really be employable, which would significantly reduce the amount of settlement they might be compelled to pay.

At their insistence, Terry agreed to be examined by a Toronto clinical neuropsychologist, Dr. Frank Kenny, for an assessment of his readiness for employment. Kenny made an extensive examination and wrote a lengthy report that was pointedly scornful of the progress that Good Sam claimed in its Evanshen file on Terry. He bluntly declared: "Vocationally, the long and the short of the matter is that it is probably not realistic to expect Mr. Evanshen to become competitively employable in the future."

Kenny added, "If he can continue to help at a clinic a few hours a week, or help coach a football team, etc., this, in addition to chores around the farm, is probably as far as things are going to go."

The insurance company, unconvinced, sought another opinion. Dr. Henry Berry, neurologist and psychiatrist, rendered it. He wrote in part, "In view of his residual deficits of memory and of other intellectual functions, along with his distractibility, limited ability to handle new and stressful situations, fatigue and vulnerability to stress, I would say that as a permanent effect of the accident and brain injury he is probably not employable in any competitive sense." That seemed to put a decisive end to the issue of Terry ever again earning a living.

Soon after Terry's arrangement in the chiropractor's clinic began, Adams made a change. He built a charming home-like office building surrounded by a treed lawn and set back from Whitby's main street. He named it the Durham Chiropractic and Rehabilitation Centre, and in the spring of 1992 he moved his practice into it. The three-storey building includes a rehabilitation gym, with such equipment as weights and a treadmill, and the building has space for two rehab therapists, two massage therapists, a naturopath, a dentist, and two chiropractors, including Adams.

The transition came just as Terry was becoming more confident of his own abilities. What Adams describes as his "aura of sadness and frustration" was lifting. Warmed by the affection and support he received from everyone at the clinic, Terry was staying longer. His stint stretched from one nervous hour to three relatively assured hours, three days a week. He was loosening up, making conversation that wasn't on his cards, and enjoying himself. His responsibilities increased to include the task of giving patients forms to fill, and escorting them on a tour of the rehab exercise room in the clinic's basement. The equipment he saw there gave him the idea of working out – in his previous life he had been a fitness enthusiast – and he joined the Whitby Recreation Centre, a health club, which he attended regularly. Terry's world was opening up.

It was to change even more. Gary Adams had long been a lecturer at the chiropractic college in Toronto, and he began to give talks as well to organizations interested in safer work places and in helping their employees avoid repetitive stress injuries. On a hunch, he asked Terry to accompany him. His only thought, a charitable one, was that it would provide Terry with an outing. Terry's role was to distribute pamphlets outlining such matters as the basic rules of posture for protecting one's spine.

"I told Terry that I would introduce him, and people could come up to chat and get the brochures," Adams says. "It turned out he liked that. He likes people. He took to it."

Terry's role expanded. He started to say a few words at the end of the chiropractor's speech. Reading from cards that he cupped in his hand, he introduced himself and explained what material he had available, and invited people to take some of it away with them.

"It was a fairly major step," Adams says, still impressed at the magnitude of the change. "I just had no idea it would go so fast for him, that he could get up and feel comfortable before a crowd of fifty, sixty people." Terry was more than comfortable. Bathed in the friendliness of a non-judgemental and attentive audience, he glowed.

Terry's success at speaking a few words at the sessions convened by Adams gave Ron Perowne, Terry's old Alouette teammate, just the opening he had been seeking. He had been nagging Terry ever since their dinner in Puyallup to give motivational addresses to high school students.

"I knew he could inspire teenagers," Perowne says. "I saw it with my own kids. Terry has charisma. He had it on the football field, where he was a megastar, and he still has it. He has the ability to hold people's attention."

At the time Perowne was working for Jostens Canada, an American company that produced graduating-class pictures and yearbooks, among such other recognition products as medals. Perowne ran the photography end of the operation in Ontario and knew he could arrange for Terry to speak in school auditoriums. His own credibility would open some doors, and most high school principals had heard of Terry Evanshen.

"He can talk about football, right?" the principals said to Perowne when he was feeling out his welcome.

"Wrong, he can't remember playing football. But he can do something better. He can talk about overcoming obstacles. Kids need to hear that."

The only hurdle remaining was to convince Terry.

Terry was horrified at the thought. For eight months he held out against Perowne's pleas, telling his friend that public speaking would be impossible for him. He would never find the right words, he would slur, he would dry, he would make a fool of himself.

"At the time I couldn't even finish a sentence, let alone a paragraph, never mind a story," Terry says. "I was stuttering within the sentences."

"Look, I'll go with you and I'll do the introduction," Perowne insisted. "Then you speak and you can read what you want to say, like you do when you go out with Gary Adams. I'll help you write it. Everyone can relate to a person who has had a hard hit in life. You've got something to give."

That last part caught Terry. He still saw himself as useless, and this was a devastating burden of shame for a proud man. And it was true that he richly enjoyed his public exposure with Gary Adams.

On April 5, 1992, the Ontario Secondary School Student Association was holding a conference titled REBEL, an acronym, at St. Patrick's high school in Toronto. Perowne was certain the name of the conference was an omen because Terry's dog was named Rebel. Perowne pays attention to omens. St. Pat's was the right place for Terry to start, he decided, and they would bring Rebel with them.

The dog was sent to the vet to be shampooed and groomed, and a ribbon was tied around his massive neck. Terry, too, was polished to a high gloss. He and Perowne wrote and rewrote a speech about the struggle of a man with no memory to put his life back together. Perowne says it contained maybe twenty-eight philosophical gems that carried the freighted messages: Don't Give Up; Believe in Yourself; Be Friendly; Family Is Important.

"It was about rising up out of the ashes," Perowne says, his eyes bright with contagious enthusiasm behind wire-rim glasses. "It was about having the hell knocked out of you, and a lot of people have been there, frankly. It was about how we need others to help us overcome challenges. We need a team, and it might be family but it might also be friends."

Terry practised the speech, pacing the living room floor, and practised it, and practised it. The plan was that Perowne would introduce him, telling students about Terry's childhood and football career and showing slides and the CFCF-TV eight-minute video Don McGowan made after the accident. Then Terry would come on stage with Rebel. Terry would open with the explanation that he would be reading the speech from the stack of cards he held in his hand, and then Rebel would withdraw to lie at the feet of Jennifer and Tara, seated in the front row.

Unexpectedly, Terry found that in front of the audience, all eyes on him, he was relaxed and even happy. The spotlight of attention felt natural and even *right*; this was how it must have been when he took a football over the goal line. "I wasn't nervous, but I was apprehensive," he explains. "I didn't want to make any mistakes, but when I got in front of those three hundred kids I was calm. The flow came easily and I felt like I was on the twenty-yard line going in to score. It was a tremendous turning point for me emotionally."

Pleased that he had taken Perowne's advice, he began, as he still does, with a curious and stilted few sentences about how *I* (he) and *you* (the audience) are going to merge into *we*. That was Perowne's suggestion to help Terry feel closer to the crowd and less isolated and self-conscious. Then Terry moved into the story of the accident, talking about his sleeplessness, his bad disposition, his inability to recognize his family, and how each day is a battle to hold himself together.

"I take — and I have to — one day at a time," Terry told the students. "I personally do not think about tomorrow. You know why? Because it doesn't belong to me. However, what I do today will influence tomorrow."

Towards the end of the speech he said touchingly, "Life is a game and you have time limits. Sometimes there's a time-out, and we know from sports that not all the players re-enter the game when the whistle blows again."

Response cards had been passed out to the three hundred teenagers in the audience. Perowne and Terry read them in the car afterwards and both men wept. One teenager wrote that her mother had just died and she didn't know how she could carry on, but hearing Terry had made her feel she could. "Why am I not a good person?" asked another. "I should love my sister more," grieved someone else, and, "I've been bad to my mother." And so on, anguished youngsters pouring out their hearts to an anguished man.

Three days later the two men spoke at another student conference, this one at St. Joseph's College in Brantford. Lorraine went to watch, finding a seat in the back row of the auditorium. She said sweetly to Perowne, "Ron, if you introduce me I'll kill you."

Perowne ignored the warning and pointed her out. After Terry's speech students crowded around him to get autographs just as they had at St. Pat's, but almost half the audience went straight to Lorraine. They wanted to know how she coped.

"She's wonderful," Perowne says. "When Terry played for the Alouettes we used to call her Minnie Max. Now I call her Saint Lorraine."

Lorraine attended Terry's speeches three more times and then quit. "I was always nervous for him, so that part was hard," she explained. "But also, I figured he's doing his thing. He's found a niche, and it's all his. I can go back now to doing my thing."

While Terry was finding his feet in high school auditoriums, another year went by with no date yet set to begin the trial that would decide how much the insurance companies would pay. This time the delay was caused by the unusual length of the trial, which was estimated to last six weeks. Trials of this length are rare for a personal injuries case, but Bernie Gluckstein expected that the two insurance companies would dispute every particular, and most especially would oppose the costs related to loss of income and Terry's future care. Finally, after many postponements, a judge had a clear enough docket to begin hearing the case, and it was set to start in November, 1993.

Gluckstein was still determined to ask the court for $2 million in damages and compensation. The insurance companies made what they said was their final offer of $1.4 million, but the Evanshens, weighing the pros and cons outlined by their lawyer, accepted Gluckstein's recommendation that they reject it.

Few cases ever have been better prepared. Mostly through the tireless and resourceful efforts of the associate lawyer on the case, Fern Silverman, folders of evidence and photographs filled eleven banker's boxes. Neuropsychologists all over the continent, the redoubtable Catherine Mateer among them, were prepared to fly to Toronto on overnight notice, their air tickets already guaranteed. A projector and screen had been prepared for the courtroom to show film of the damaged Jeep and of Terry playing football. Teammates from across the country were ready to come to Toronto. Tracy, Tara, and Jennifer had written compelling accounts of their difficult lives with their altered father. The first witnesses would be Terry, Lorraine, the three daughters, Terry's mother, and two of Terry's brothers, Frank and Fred. Gluckstein and Fern Silverman had briefed them all on courtroom protocol. Two witnesses to the accident were standing by. Durham police constable Chuck Nash was prepared to appear. People who had worked with Terry in his former sales jobs were awaiting their turn to be called. Coaches from the Alouettes, Tiger-Cats, and Argonauts would also be witnesses. Doctors by the half dozen would testify about Terry's brain injuries, and Barry Brown, a Toronto family mediator, was ready to describe the shattered state of the Evanshen family relationships and social life.

Gluckstein believed that the trial would cost the plaintiff more than a hundred thousand dollars just to pay travel and hotel costs and the expert-witness fees.

Gluckstein had fat, indexed, loose-leaf binders assembled by Silverman, a forthright, clear-headed woman, to guide him through the maze. His opening address to the jury was written, but he knew it so well the outline would serve merely as an occasional reference. He felt great confidence. His experts not only outnumbered the defendants' lawyers two to one, but in almost every case they were much better qualified. And he knew that Terry's confused state of mind would inevitably emerge during his testimony, the best evidence the jury would have of the wreckage of his brain.

Gluckstein and Silverman drove separately to the Evanshen farm on Saturday, two days before the trial, to make a final "prep" of the Evanshens. It is unethical to tell witnesses what they should say in their testimony but lawyers customarily take time to orient them to the arcane procedures of a courtroom and such matters as how to address the judge.

Events were moving rapidly. The lawyer for the insurance company holding coverage for the man who caused the accident suddenly declared that his client was willing to settle out of court for $500,000, the maximum allowed in the policy's coverage. That was acceptable to the Evanshens and their lawyers, which left Terry's insurance company alone on the field. Several times on Saturday and again early the next day, Silverman spoke with Darcy Duke, the lawyer representing Terry's insurance company and a glum man known to associates as "the dark prince." His client was trying to avoid parting with the million dollars that was the limit in Terry's policy. The exchanges were so urgent that a few times Silverman was negotiating from a phone booth.

On Sunday afternoon, Silverman returned to the Evanshen farm to make sure everyone there felt prepared for the ordeal ahead. She found Ron Perowne there. He had dropped in to share his apprehensions about his imminent court appearance on Terry's behalf. After reassuring them all, Silverman left the farm early that afternoon to drive to Bernie Gluckstein's home, where she would go over final details with him and connect with Darcy Duke one last time. Late in the afternoon, Duke offered her a pleasant surprise. Feeling exposed by the withdrawal of the other insurance company, his client wished to settle. Would the Evanshens accept $1 million, the policy limit, with a sweetener on the offer of an additional one hundred thousand?

That made a total settlement of $1.6 million. Gluckstein still thought it was low, but Silverman disagreed. In any case, it was up to the Evanshens to decide. Silverman phoned the Evanshens to tell them the proposal.

"I think it is the best we can get," she said frankly.

Lorraine and Terry were heartily sick of the five-year-long litigation process. They spent almost no time at all deciding to take the offer.

The $1.6 million payment was widely publicized, and seemed to most people to be a luxurious sum, but the facts of the situation were vastly different. The Evanshens paid Gluckstein $200,000, an amount that probably was much less than the case cost his firm. Then they paid the money owed to Epson, Terry's former employer, a debt that had been running up interest and amounted to about $160,000. They owed their bank almost $200,000 on the line of credit, and the insurance companies deducted from the settlement the substantial advance payments Gluckstein had compelled them to make. At the end of the day, Terry wound up with about $400,000.

It was some time before payment was forthcoming because Gluckstein's firm was breaking up and its accounts were in somewhat of a jumble. A troubleshooter, Don McIntyre, an astute man in his mid-thirties, was hired to straighten out the confusion, and he promptly cleared the cheque for the Evanshens. He did something else. An avid golfer who now owns the Pines of Georgia Golf Club near Lake Simcoe, he decided Terry should play golf.

"Have you ever golfed?" he asked.

"I think so," Terry replied, recalling that golf clubs were stored somewhere in the farmhouse.

"Good," said McIntyre. "We'll have a game."

Terry was alarmed on two counts. One was that he would be as inept at hitting a golf ball as he had been initially at catching a football, and the other, more serious concern, was that golf is a game ill-suited to a man who can't control his temper.

"There is no way I can play golf," Terry thought to himself. "I don't have the temperament to be patient."

He tried explaining to McIntyre that golf was not for him, but the man wouldn't listen. Besides, Terry was intrigued by the prospect of playing a competitive game again. And Lorraine said merrily, "Don, if you'll take him off my hands for an afternoon, I'll pay you." McIntyre booked a tee-off time and Terry nervously stepped up to the ball. He hit it poorly but the line of his body when he swung was unmistakably that of a good golfer. On that first round McIntyre watched Terry struggle to regain the honed coordination golf requires, and decided that he only needed practice to become a fine player again.

"He's a very competitive person," McIntyre notes, "so he had a lot of frustration in the beginning, but I never saw him really blow up. And he wants to learn. He's like my twelve-year-old son. He keeps asking what he is doing wrong, and what he needs to do to improve." McIntyre adds, "Terry is a wonderful human being. He's a very caring, loving person."

Terry is now a member of McIntyre's golf club, where he holds a respectable 18 handicap.

Relying on advice from their bank, the Canadian Imperial Bank of Commerce, and its financial arm, Wood Gundy, Terry and Lorraine shrewdly invested what was left of the insurance company's settlement and tried to live on the interest. They allowed themselves only one luxury, the purchase of a two-week time-share apartment in Aruba, right on a beach of fine white sand lapped by the blue Caribbean Sea.

On their first holiday there, when no witnesses were around, Tara and Jennifer taught their father to swim in a pool on the property. He had been avoiding water, chagrined that he couldn't swim. He was greatly humiliated that he had to learn as a toddler does, with the girls supporting his tummy in the shallow end, and exhorting him to kick. "Basically, I learned to dog-paddle," he admits sheepishly. "I was so embarrassed. You have no idea how frustrating it was. I called myself a dingbat and a moron a thousand times." But he now can swim the length of a small pool, although with much splashing.

Lorraine was pleased for him but what had begun as an annoyance was assuming major proportions in her mind. Terry's inability to be a social person with his family was becoming hard to take. She understood to a degree his restless pursuit of activity, but she longed for quiet companionship. She found that Terry could supply conviviality only on demand. Even when he pulled up a chair at her request and tried to engage in the usual marital small-talk, he did so with an edginess that suggested he was needed elsewhere for something much more important, like putting wood chips around the bases of the apple trees.

When asked why it never occurred to him to have lazy time with his family, his expression went blank. "I have no idea," he answered.

Terry understood Lorraine's needs when they were explained to him, but he couldn't originate a warm response spontaneously and Lorraine felt humiliated to have to ask him for friendship. In turn, he was dismayed on those occasions when she lost patience and charged him with insensitivity.

Their disputes were disconcerting for both of them. Terry needs peace of mind in order to keep his fragile thought processes from shattering, so when he and Lorraine have a sharp exchange, he almost cannot function. Bewildered and confused, his concentration falls into total disorder. If he is driving some-where after a dispute with his wife, he needs a list of every part of the route because his uncertain ability to hold a memory breaks down completely. At those times he is also more vulnerable if something unexpected happens. Terry can feel himself becoming what he calls "rougher." His voice becomes loud as he moves into unbridled wrath. He knows he is accelerating into a tantrum but he can't stop. He no longer has control of what will happen next.

Good Sam taught him that he should walk away at the first sign of irritation, but he can rarely do that before his anger erupts. After that, he can't stop himself from ranting. "There's no shut-off button," he explains unhappily.

During his daily "naps," Terry reviews the most recent loss of control and hates himself. But since he knows that the last thing he needs is to use this important rest period to berate himself, he tries diversion. The most peaceful distraction in his repertoire is a mental picture of himself walking on a beach. He summons that to mind, but after an outburst or a quarrel with Lorraine it doesn't work. He can't stop brooding about his failures. "Why didn't I do this?" he asks himself. "Why did I do that?"

That same spring of 1993 saw a change in their household. Tracy Lee, now twenty-three, moved out to share an apartment with Joe Clark, her boyfriend of about five years. Terry's mother, Aline, took over the vacated bedroom, which Lorraine redecorated invitingly to please her.

Aline had been living with one or another of her many chil-dren ever since John Evanshen's death in 1982. Her most recent residence had been with her son Gordon in Toronto, but when his marriage broke up, the house was sold as part of the marital property split. Gordon had moved into a place too small to accommodate his mother.

Aline's relocation to live with Terry and Lorraine seemed a sensible one, since there was an empty bedroom and Lorraine could use Aline's help with Terry. Lorraine assumed, in any case, that the arrangement was temporary and she expected that Aline would do as she had been doing for ten years, which was to live for a few months or years at a time with a few of her children in turn. But somehow time went by and Aline remained with Terry and Lorraine, paying occasional short visits to her son Frank in Vancouver or her daughter Barbara, an industrious woman with a prosperous berry farm in Scotland. Lorraine and Aline had a fairly easy relationship and the Brooklin farmhouse held many comforts for Aline, not the least of which was its proximity to Casino Rama, a gambling centre near Orillia, where she delighted in pitting her old age pension against the vagaries of slot machines.

Meanwhile, Lorraine suffered two hard blows. In the fall of 1993, her sister Allison died, and this was followed two years later by the death of another sister, Pat.

With Aline in the house to help watch over Terry, Lorraine thought the time was right for her to go back to paid employment and boost the family income. When she broached the subject, however, she was met with a wall of opposition. Terry was adamant that Lorraine stay home, and Jennifer, fifteen at the time, protested that she wanted Lorraine there when she arrived back from school. Lorraine dropped the idea.

The Canadian Football League paid Terry a handsome tribute in November 1994, when it named a trophy for him. The award for the most outstanding player in the Eastern Division "possessing the highest qualities of courage, fair play, and sportsmanship" had been known as the Jeff Russel Memorial Trophy for the gentlemanly quarterback who played at the beginning of the century, but the Russel family asked that the name be withdrawn. The announcement of the name change referred to Terry's "tremendous accomplishments on the playing field."

Curiously, the Evanshens haven't heard a word about the award since. They are never invited to the presentation and, judging by the annual awards list, Terry's name has disappeared from the trophy.

Family responsibilities and the high overhead of running the farm began cast a different light on Terry's lectures to teenagers. What had started as a therapeutic diversion for him began to look like a serious source of needed income. Every neuropsychologist's report of Terry's employment possibilities had used some form of the phrase "unfit for *competitive* employment," but speech-making is not a competitive activity in the same sense as meeting a sales quota. Indeed, in 1993 one of Terry's many examiners, Toronto neurologist W.J. McIlroy, had anticipated such an occupation for him. Commenting on the studies that ruled out Terry ever functioning in a competitive environment, McIlroy wrote, "This is not an all-or-nothing situation. . . . I feel that with sufficient motivation he would be capable of handling a non-stressful routine work environment."

Terry was finding speech-making anything but stressful. The right word for his emotion on a platform might even be exhilaration, and he was getting better and better at performing. He and Perowne frequently were accorded standing ovations, and appreciative letters poured in after every presentation – the words "profound," "inspiring," "moving," and "outstanding" occur frequently among the accolades.

Their speaking circuit had broadened over two years from school auditoriums, where the fee was fifty dollars, or sometimes nothing, to appearances in posh hotels before sales meetings of large corporations, where they might receive hundreds of dollars. With Ron doing the bookings, they extended themselves beyond Ontario, appearing in Calgary, Montreal, Lennoxville, Baltimore, and Vancouver. Perowne was no longer at Jostens, and was relying instead on odd jobs for the CFL, so he too was interested in turning speech-making into a lucrative career.

They formed themselves into a company, *Speaking for Life*, whose failure to prosper was of spectacular proportions. Perowne still has a bank statement, and not an exceptional one, which shows the firm's balance at $29.75. The problem was that Perowne was constitutionally incapable of hustling for bookings or asking people to pay even a reasonable professional fee. For the CFL's Stay in School campaign, for instance, they spoke free. For a while, the Ontario Head Injury Association collaborated as a sponsor, but this relationship didn't last. Perowne looked to the banks for sponsorship, but disgustedly found his efforts were futile. He still believes nobly that what Terry does is a form of public service, but he couldn't sell that concept to anyone.

Perowne was tiring. Despite his unflagging affection and admiration for Terry, escorting him had proved to be very labour intensive. Besides organizing the administrative details surrounding each presentation, Perowne had to protect Terry from becoming agitated before his speech, or else he would fall apart. Terry's sudden flashes of rage meant that Perowne had to learn how to soothe him so that Terry would be socially presentable. Also, Terry's high level of anxiety was exasperating for his collaborator: forgetting he had already been told the answer, Terry would ask over and over if Perowne had attended to their audio requirements, or if the motel reservation had been confirmed.

One morning he and Terry were driving by a handsome high school in Aurora, north of Toronto. "That's a good-looking school," Terry said to Perowne. "Maybe we should speak there."

Perowne replied evenly, "We did. Yesterday."

With his wife, Gail, headed for law school, Perowne had to face the inescapable fact that he needed permanent employment. He was unhappy to inform Terry that their relationship would have to end. Both men were deeply distressed at the prospect of parting, but just at that critical point, Ann Firstbrook came into Terry's life. In December 1994, Ann's husband, John Firstbrook, who works in life insurance, heard Terry speak at a gathering sponsored by a brain injury association. John came home raving to his wife about Terry's amazing power to hold the room in the palm of his hand. Impressed, he arranged for Ron and Terry to speak at two meetings of underwriters, one a breakfast in a Toronto hotel that same month and the other a conference in Orlando, Florida, in January. Ann, by coincidence, was making travel arrangements for both events.

Ann Firstbrook, a slender, gracious, cultivated woman then in her thirties, was having difficulty finding her place in the world of paid work. The only daughter of a demanding man, she has suffered intermittent bouts of severe depression during a career that has encompassed being a ski instructor in Vermont, running a fitness institute, and fundraising for the Heart Foundation. After her marriage she was often needed at home to nurse John, who broke his neck in a diving accident when he was eighteen and has had nine serious operations on his disintegrating spine since then.

At the time that Terry's speech impressed her husband, Ann had just been pushed out of a travel agency she helped start, one that arranged the bonus trips that some companies offer their star employees. She turned next to being an independent travel broker, occasionally hiring speakers for corporate events, which is how she happened to be involved in underwriters' gatherings in Toronto and Orlando. When she contacted Ron Perowne to discuss travel details, she was surprised to learn that he was asking the fee of fifteen hundred dollars for them both, which Ann knew was well below the norm for a star draw.

"He saw those speeches as Terry's rehabilitation," Ann explains. "The money part didn't come easily to him. Ron is the kindest person you'll ever meet and he has been a real true friend to Terry."

When she called to book the charter flight tickets for Orlando, Ann knew only that Perowne and Terry were former football players and she envisioned them as hulks. She was exasperated when the airline would not allow her to select their seats. "These are *football players*," she told the agent indignantly. "They are the size of refrigerators. You'll have to give me aisle seats."

At her husband's insistence, Ann attended the breakfast meeting in Toronto to hear them speak. When she saw Terry and Perowne, both of them five foot ten when they stretch their necks, her first thought was, "Thank God. They'll fit in middle seats."

Terry sat beside her at breakfast and she was moved by his shyness. His expression, as Ann describes it, was that of "a lost lamb."

"Terry," she said as an ice-breaker, "I've heard great things about you."

Terry gravely told her that he had fumbled only three times in his entire fourteen-year career. That startled her but she was touched by the intensity of his attention on her. "When he was looking at me, he actually focussed on looking at me, and he seemed sincerely interested in what I was saying," she recalls. Unaware that Terry must concentrate deeply in every conversation in order to follow it, she thought only that he was an exceedingly polite man.

When she mentioned that she was making his travel arrangements to Orlando, Terry brightened. "Ronnie is thinking of doing something else soon. What do you think about the two of us working together?" he asked her impulsively.

She didn't see how she could say no. "Well," she said cautiously, "why don't we try it for six months?" Terry let out a sigh of relief and gratitude.

A few minutes later when she heard Terry speak, he touched her own depth of sorrow. His struggle also mirrored her husband's game battle to keep going despite constant back pain. "This guy tries so hard," she thought compassionately of Terry. "Anybody who is trying that hard to come back from a bad blow deserves whatever help I can give."

But she still had second thoughts about the arrangement which she had taken on so impetuously. "What have I done?" she asked herself. "I'm busy enough already. I don't really need this."

That morning she spent about an hour on the phone to some of her contacts in the business world, and in no time at all had a modest but not inconsiderable list of bookings for Terry's "motivational speech" at a better fee than Terry and Perowne had ever commanded together. Amazed, she decided she just might have a productive new sideline.

Ann made some changes. Without Perowne to provide Terry's background in his twenty-minute introduction, Terry's speech would have to expand beyond its former twenty minutes to include the biographical elements. Ann had noted the questions people asked after the speech and she helped Terry incorporate information she thought would cover some points about which audiences seemed confused. She also suggested he downplay his football career, and drew from him and Lorraine stories he might use instead: about the time he almost drowned, his tenure at the chiropractic clinic that helped him get back into society, and waking his children to walk with him at two in the morning.

"What he added was more of the process he went through – is still going through," she explains. "We just filled in more details."

Their arrangement from the beginning was that Ann would find the clients, set the fee (usually five thousand dollars a speech plus expenses), draw up a contract, make the arrangements, and also – as it turned out – travel with Terry for forty percent of the fee, out of which she pays all promotion and business expenses.

The new partnership was launched in March 1995, just after Terry's return from the family's annual visit to their time-share apartment in Aruba, where he had picked up a becoming tan. Terry, drenched in apprehension, practiced his forty-five minute speech for days in advance of his first booking, but found as soon as he moved to the microphone that he was just fine working alone. The buoyant feeling he had when he and Ron Perowne faced an audience was still there for him as the solo speaker.

The speech, titled "Seize Each Day," is printed in large letters on 102 square cardboard cards of a size Terry can hold comfortably in his hand, and key words are highlighted in yellow so he can pick them out with a downward glance. Nervous that he might some day drop the bulky stack of cards in the middle of the speech, he has numbered each one on both sides to make it easier for him to reassemble them quickly in the right order.

Five years later, after giving that speech about forty times a year, he still didn't have it memorized. In fact, when asked to present it without the cards, he could only stumble through a sentence or two. "I am going to tell you about my two lives," he said, and then trailed off. "Before and after," he was prompted. He picked it up. "Before and after a car collision and I'll refer to them as my first and second lives . . ." He faltered again, and threw up his hands.

Ann thinks she was more worried than he when Terry went to the podium for the first time. Foremost in her mind was that he was brain-injured, and she should not expect normalcy. She was not surprised when he told her that he could not speak on two consecutive days. Given his limited stamina, it made sense to her. Only months later did she learn that the reason he didn't want to speak two days in a row was because he didn't like to shave two days in a row. His skin is so sensitive it is irritated by daily shaves.

"Terry, I gotta tell you, get with it," she told him, taking off the kid gloves. "If I can get you two engagements in two days, you're doing them. Buy some face cream."

Ann was dismayed at Terry's behaviour the first time a sponsor wanted to meet Terry before making a decision to hire him as a speaker. Terry was so intimidated by the situation that he scarcely could open his mouth. "There I was pushing that he's a charismatic, inspirational speaker," she says, shaking her head ruefully, "and there he was – completely withdrawn."

Terry got over that with time and became assured and charming when required to present himself for viewing. What didn't change, however, was something Ann was slow to realize. Terry is at his worst on Fridays. He is not certain of the explanation himself, whether it is because two relatively empty weekend days are ahead of him and he abhors the prospect of unregulated time, or whether he is plain tired from a four-day stretch of concentrating every minute on what he is doing and what he is saying. On Fridays he even finds it difficult even to follow his routine, and the extra mental effort he must exert makes him uncommunicative. Ann learned to steer clear of Friday meetings with sponsors when she could, but she accepted Friday bookings to speak and just hoped for the best.

The routine that filled Terry's mornings six days a week at that time was a rigid one that postponed for him the overwhelming stress of unstructured time. At six-thirty each morning at the farm, the alarm wakened him from his fitful sleep. He dressed, plugged in the coffee maker, which had been set up the night before, and shaved. He gave a cookie to his dog Simba, a shaggy white Great Pyrenees, and then walked to the mailbox at the end of the driveway, eating a banana on the way, and got the newspaper. While sipping his coffee he leafed through the sports section, and then he picked up his gym bag, which he had packed the night before with clean clothes. Climbing into the Jeep, he drove eight kilometres to the Whitby Recreational Club for his three-hour workout while eating another banana.

"Once I'm in that gym, I'm in another world," Terry says. First he did stretching exercises. Then on Mondays and Thursdays he worked on his shoulders; Tuesdays and Fridays were chest days, and Wednesdays and Saturdays were legs days. This daunting routine was modified somewhat in the fall of 1999, but only because Terry dislocated his shoulder and was told that his work-outs were too strenuous for a battered man in his fifties. His concession to his aging frame was to cut the routines back an hour and drop the Saturday one.

He continues this regimen to this day. Invariably, though, when he returns home from the gym, he walks Simba. He steps out briskly, arms swinging, in the way he developed when his balance was poor and his crippled right arm needed stretching. Then, around eleven, he has what he calls brunch, cereal and vitamins, and maybe toast. He prepares this himself because he detests feeling dependent on others, but if Lorraine makes him something more substantial he'll eat it. That does him until dinner, except for the handfuls of candy he eats in his car.

With that comfortingly repetitious start, Terry is ready to leave the farm and enter into the unsettling world of variables where the unexpected might happen and he can't foresee how he will react. When his schedule permits, he likes to postpone the exposure to embarrassment as long as possible. One device is to tackle farm chores. He inspects the fences for breaks, prepares the horse feed and water, and always double-checks the latches on the stalls, because so often he has forgotten to do that.

Nothing he does is automatic and performed without think-ing about it, as people do when they drive a familiar route, their minds on something else. Terry has to think his way through each errand, muttering to himself, "Pay attention. Concentrate." He still keeps a Daytimer in the car but he no longer has to consult it constantly unless his concentration is interrupted. If he is distracted by something unexpected, he has to check the book before he can resume his schedule.

As his speaking career burgeoned in the nineties, a part of one or two days a week was to drive to the spanking new house in north Toronto where Ann and John Firstbrook live with their newly adopted Russian-born son, Andrew. The trips were more to pass the time than for any urgent business, but Terry and Ann would discuss such matters as setting up the Terry Evanshen Web site, or go over a new brochure to advertize his availability as a speaker. Then he would drive back to the farm, able to drive from memory without looking at a map. Once there, he immediately looked for another task to occupy himself.

In the first two years of Terry's partnership with Ann, while bookings built up slowly, Ann kept working as a freelance travel agent, but in 1997 Terry had become so popular on the speakers' circuit that she dropped everything else to devote herself exclusively to his flourishing career.

In those early years Ann found some aspects of Terry's memory problems hard to bear. The example she gives is the time when her father had a heart attack. She told Terry about it and he expressed concern, but the next few times she saw him he talked about himself and didn't inquire how her father was doing. She thought he was being insensitive until she realized that he had forgotten that her father was ill.

Terry's temper came as another shock. "He can get angry in an instant, and it is not a pretty anger," she says. "He can get all the way to rage very quickly." In their first year of working together she would yell back and she estimates that Terry stormed out of her office one in every three meetings. Then she learned that when Terry did something annoying, such as keeping her waiting two hours for a meeting, she could tell him frankly that his behaviour was inconsiderate, but she had better not blow up. Terry can't abide people raising their voices to him. To avoid his father's tantrums, Terry as a child escaped by plunging into sports. Before the accident, he used the same escape tactic whenever Lorraine was angry with him: he simply left the room. For a man who could not remember much, certain of his former coping mechanisms seemed to be indelible.

Many of Terry's early speaking engagements were in the Toronto area, which made it easy for Ann to attend. Other times Ann had a reason to go with him to the event because of some other involvement, so it wasn't immediately apparent to her that travelling everywhere with Terry would be a permanent part of the package. She soon discovered that, left to himself, Terry is a loose cannon. The problem was not so much that Terry could get easily lost or confused, though those were real obstacles in the beginning. Experience eventually enabled Terry to be confident enough in airports to find the departure gate or taxi stand, though often he doesn't know what city he is in, and time-zone changes baffle him. The larger issue was his ungovernable hair-trigger temper. He would blast a hotel employee for mixing up his reservation, or yell at a sponsor who was late meeting the plane. Ann's job description soon included staying at Terry's side to protect him from annoyances that would cause his charm to slip. Especially, she never left him alone with clients.

"In this business, not everything goes smoothly," she explained in the midst of a busy period of speeches in the summer of 1999, "and you have to ride with the aggravations. Terry can't do that." She ran interference to make sure Terry didn't "get ticked off, because the last thing an audience wants is an uptight, crabby speaker. And word-of-mouth can hurt you. When I'm there, my job is to make it easy for Terry to be the nice guy he really is."

Terry doesn't dispute this view of his behaviour. "Little things get blown into big things," he confesses with regret. "I lose my concentration, which I must have to do the speech. So I really do need someone to take care of everything."

Since the sponsor had the unusual expense of paying for two tickets to get one speaker, Terry and Ann usually flew economy class whenever Terry was booked to give a speech out of town. Ann would act as a guard to intervene when irritants threatened to destabilize him. She says that if flight attendants didn't let him hang his suit bag in the executive-class closet, he went "ballistic, because he doesn't want his clothes to wrinkle." She would talk him down, and sometimes she used humour. "These seats are really narrow," he groused one day, beginning to steam. "So what," she said airily. "You're just a little guy." He was amused and his anger vanished.

"I joke with him, I kid him constantly," Ann explained one day in the spring of 1999 as she was checking some brochures. "And I tell him when he's driving me nuts. But his idiosyncrasies don't bug me any more. He never says, 'Poor me.' He never does that. He's not a depressing person to be around."

Whenever Terry rambled, as always happens when he tires, Ann usually paid no attention, but sometimes she would interrupt crisply, "Terry, you're all over the place."

He would reply quietly, touchingly, "I know."

Almost unconsciously, she learned not to tell Terry more than a few things at once. A long recital of arrangements would cause him to stop trying to remember any of it. "If you say ten things to me," he confessed to her, "it doesn't register at all."

As part of the protective wall she put around Terry before a speech, Ann made certain that no media interviews or social gatherings were scheduled for him in the period before he was due on the platform. The energy required to answer reporters' questions or engage in chit-chat with sponsors would leave him too drained to give the speech.

"My job is to keep him focussed, and not let him get agitated," she explained. A fixed part of this protection was to assure Terry of an hour or so of solitude in his hotel room or a private space backstage before an appearance. Terry used the quiet time to go over the speech aloud maybe twice, shuffling the 102 cards deftly, and then he would lie on a bed or cot to rest his faculties; his favourite technique was to imagine himself walking on a deserted beach. With about a half-hour to go, he would rise and groom himself. He put on his trousers last thing, just before leaving the room, and would not sit down until the speech was done. That preserves the crease.

After the speech, when people lined up to talk to Terry or get his autograph, Ann performed two useful functions. As best she could, she kept the interchanges one-on-one. Terry can't divide his attention in order to respond to more than one person at a time. She also gauged how much stamina he had left in him after the speech, drawing him away from the lineup with some excuse when she saw him flagging.

"He has about two hours of intensity in him," Ann explains, "and after that he is wiped. He starts talking in circles. Ask him about the accident and he'll answer with a football story or tell you how they found their farm."

Ann watched for the inevitable moment after a speech when Terry couldn't follow a question and wouldn't admit he'd lost it.

If he launched into the anecdote about how he was inspired by Nolan Ryan when he had been asked about his fitness program, Ann would touch his arm lightly and say, "I don't mean to interrupt, Terry, but . . ." People who didn't know the situation would be affronted on his behalf, thinking her overbearing, but Terry always gave her an understanding and grateful glance. "He's great that way," Ann said. "For everyone else it is rude as hell, but he's fine with that." Ann found that Terry's vitality would be restored afterwards by a half-hour or so of withdrawal in his room.

Ann always said to him just before his speech, "Go out there and have fun," but light humour was not in his emotional vocabulary until almost ten years after the accident. Gradually, as his confidence improved, Terry loosened up enough to be dryly humorous. "In questions and answers he can be really funny," Ann says. Once, when he was asked if he lost his driver's licence after the accident, he replied with a chuckle that no, he didn't lose his ability to drive. "But I drive at about sixty K on the highways with people honking at me. None of my family wants to drive with me." That got a laugh of recognition in which Terry joined, looking like a mischievous child.

When Lorraine met Ann she liked her "right off the bat." Lorraine saw her as a partner. "She deals with Terry's ups and downs in his business life, and I deal with his ups and down at home. We have a lot in common."

Lorraine adds with a whoop of laughter, "And I was glad to get rid of him."

Terry counted Lorraine, and then Ann, as the two people most important to the level of functioning he had achieved by the late 1990s. "I need that direction," he explained in the somewhat jumbled fashion that marks his discourse. "Once I get on stage,

I'm in my own world, but to get to that stage there's a lot of pieces that have to be put together. Lorraine covers all the stability and everything else in my real life of home and once I've got to get out to the real world, society, well then for me to be at my best I need some direction."

He has no difficulty at all relying on women to help him, or in admitting he needs their help. A woman friend wondered about him, a jock to his toes, surrounded by women and acknowledging his dependency on them. He explained, sort of. "If I need to ask you for your help, you know I'm asking from my heart," he said earnestly. "And I will know immediately if you're receiving it in the same text and visa versa." The syntax is scrambled, but his drift is clear: if he trusts someone — man or woman — he doesn't question their motives.

Terry has been working his way to this softer version of himself ever since the accident, and the long learning curve has been worth it. Magic happens when Terry Evanshen gives a speech. He is fascinating on a platform. He paces, as graceful and edgy as a cat, and is compellingly intense and focussed on what he is saying. He is so hypnotic that his sidelong peeks at the cards cupped in his hand are almost unnoticeable. Handsome, trim, and iron-muscled from his workouts, he wears the best tailoring and gleams with health. Though he is in his mid-fifties, his face is unlined and his jawline is as taut as a thirty-year-old's. The packaging is impressive enough, but the content is heart-stirring and unforgettable. Terry is touchingly open and vulnerable as he describes the grief of living with deep damage to his memory, and his daily struggle to be proud of himself. It touches a place in most people's souls: loss and self-doubt are the common currency of everyone's reality.

Ron Perowne often speaks of Terry's charisma, which Ann Firstbrook calls his *persona*. "He gets up there on the platform and just shows himself," she says. "His story is pretty extraordinary, but he reaches people most with his honesty. He's touchable. Audiences connect with him, and no one is afraid to approach him after the speech."

That non-judgemental approval has done more to heal Terry Evanshen than all his years of therapy. He explains, "Over the last couple of years, I think the kind of responses I'm getting from people is giving me another purpose. A fulfilment. I just say to myself, 'I must have been an entertainer in my first life, and I must have been a good one, but I know I'm touching people's hearts now.' So I don't think I suffered any loss in that accident. I gained a heck of a lot."

That's Terry at his bravest, but some days he can't pull it off. Once Terry asked Ann Firstbrook to read a social worker's report that he had just received. It gave a stark picture of his prospects, with a list of the searing limitations that he could expect to exist for the rest of his life. As she read it, dismayed, Terry said, "This is what I am left with. This is my soul."

In 1995, Toronto's Clarke Institute of Psychiatry presented Terry with its Courage to Come Back Award.

T E N

What's in Terry Evanshen's head? Usually he can't carry anything more than whatever he is doing at the moment; his brain cannot handle much else. He can't process what to do about a problem with his car while shovelling snow. In 1985, Dr. Endel Tulving, a pre-eminent memory researcher now at the Rotman Research Institute in Toronto, reported on a patient very much like Terry, a man with profound amnesia who could remember nothing from his past or imagine his future. He was left in what Tulving described as a state of "permanent present," which is Terry's fate.

Terry's brain sustained many kinds of damage, but most of his malfunctions seem to relate to his frontal lobes, which somehow act as the window on old memories and enable multiple tasking. While he has shown heroic adaptation to his inability to split his concentration, the absence of his past has been crippling. Because Terry cannot recall more than a glimmer of his first forty-four years, he can't project himself into the future and he hasn't been able to fully regain his old personality. The enthusiasm of his old self, the warm responsiveness he acquired over his formative years, the tolerance for setbacks that he learned, with difficulty, are returning only minutely. He wants the self-control, tact, spontaneity and conviviality that once were his, but they haven't yet emerged.

What he misses least, because it is for him unimaginable, is the ability everyone older than a young child has, which is to think about the future. In order to picture what he will do next weekend, or decide to try something new, he would need to know himself. He requires self-awareness, which would be his if he could harvest the experiences of his first lifetime. Then he could mentally test which possible scenarios would suit the wide range of capabilities known to him. Terry cannot project his self into tomorrow because he has only a small piece of his self. The bridges to his deeper identity are gone.

One scientist described the simultaneous process of using the past in order to imagine how something will go tomorrow as "memories of the future."

In the Middle Ages, Boncompagno da Signa, the sage of Bologna, described memory as "a glorious and admirable gift of nature by which we recall past things, we embrace present things, and we contemplate future things *through their likeness to past things.*"

Awareness of oneself, which Terry has in very limited supply, is a construct dependent on the brain being able to gather up the pieces of identity with which old memories are drenched. Human behaviour is an amalgam of life lessons that swirl in the unconscious and shape present responses. Terry Evanshen, who has no supportive memory of his first four decades, operates instead on the wistful hope that what he is now constructing will one day be a whole person functioning normally. Meanwhile he balances on a high wire. The safety net of life-experience continuity available to people without brain injuries does not exist for him.

"You have to begin to lose your memory, if only in bits and pieces, to realize that memory is what makes our lives," wrote film director Luis Buñuel, "Life without memory is no life at all. . . . Without it, we are nothing."

Esther Salaman, in her book *A Collection of Memories*, wrote of "the sacred and precious memories of childhood" and how ungrounded and bankrupt life is without them. Commenting on this observation, Oliver Sacks added, "an ultimate serenity and security of spirit [in old age] is only given to those who possess, or recall, the true past."

It is old news that memory and a sense of one's identity are inseparable. Such sages as the philosopher William James described the integration, but only lately has there begun an understanding of where — though not how — the brain does it. What emerged in the nineties, which the United States Congress declared the Decade of the Brain, was the beginning of an understanding of the brain's anatomy. Technology now permits neuroscientists to watch blood moving in a living brain, and they are able to make some assumptions about the brain's engineering. They can't yet *see* memory, but they have learned that it is not a location but a circuitry.

Dr. Donald T. Stuss, the neuropsychologist who is director of the prestigious Rotman Research Institute in Toronto, is one of the major figures on the frontier of neuroscience. Stuss is a balding, friendly man with a nose pleasantly off-centre who has the gifts of patience and clarity found in born teachers. In fact he was a high school teacher of Latin in the 1950s, at the time of the Hall-Dennis report, which ushered in an era of structureless classrooms and curricula. Stuss believed that Emmett Hall, later a judge on Canada's Supreme Court, and Lloyd Dennis, an education reformer, had committed a pedagogical error. Stuss was convinced that children learn best when the environment is orderly. He was so intrigued by the mystery of cognitive development that he set about gaining an education in neuropsychology, an emerging field, and this put him on a path to becoming what he is now, a world leader in the neurosciences.

In March 2000 he co-chaired an international conference in Toronto that was devoted exclusively to the latest findings about frontal lobes and brought together the foremost frontal-lobe researchers in the world to decide the course of future exploration. In impenetrable jargon they excitedly told one another they now know a lot about frontal lobes and, also, they still don't know much. No one, for instance, knows how to *fix* lobe damage.

This is hardly surprising. Serious research into frontal and temporal lobes, and why memory loss occurs when they are damaged, is only a few decades old, although advances are proceeding at a galloping pace. The investigations are fuelled by the new technology and by the increasing availability of generous research grants to study Alzheimer's disease, whose incidence has increased sharply as people in developed countries live longer than their parents did.

Eleven years after Terry's accident, his neurologist, Doug Waller, requested an MRI in order to ascertain just what had happened in Terry's brain. The result raised almost as many questions as it answered. Waller explained, "There are hundreds of thousands of pathways and some of these areas are shrunken. We can see the white matter has atrophied but we don't know what is gone. We can only say something has happened."

The test did confirm what Waller believed from the beginning – that the bump on the head Terry suffered was the least of his brain's damage. "We wanted to know if there were signs of bleeding trauma. Pulped brains swell, but we didn't see that much on the CT scans and the MRI confirmed that there had been little bleeding inside the skull. We have to conclude that the most serious injuries occurred because Terry's brain was suffocated."

Waller was interested to note evidence in the MRI analysis that, in a sense, holes were punched in the white matter of Terry's brain. "That explains why he has some things working, like his coordination, while other things adjacent to the centres for coordination are gone." The most likely explanation for the loss of Terry's past is the diffuse axonal injury together with oxygen deprivation, and maybe a concordant reduction of blood flow, the condition known as hypoxic-ischemic injury. The combination knocked out old-memory linkage all over his brain.

Terry's brain may still contain some of his past memories, lodged in neurons no longer in touch with one another because of axon damage. Don Stuss once knew a man who lost his entire past for a short while and then, suddenly, everything flooded back. The pathways had repaired themselves. Since Terry's pre-accident memories had not returned more than a decade later, chances are, unhappily, that they never will.

Occasionally pieces of flotsam bob up in Terry's seamless sea. He can't summon up a scene in the classroom of his high school, or a New Year's Eve party in Calgary, or revisit in his mind his successful selling trip to Europe, but he has flashes of recognition about the *look* of places. Once when approaching Montreal by train he was staring out the window as the junk-filled backyards of Pointe St-Charles slid by, and he said idly, "That's where I used to play. We stole fruit from those trees." Who was with him when he stole apples? He doesn't know. They are not in his picture.

One Thanksgiving weekend while strolling in Montreal, he directed his family unerringly to a shortcut; Lorraine and Tara stared at one another in amazement.

Another time, entering Nick's Steak House across from Calgary's McMahon Stadium, he knew he had been there before. He was right. It was, in fact, a haunt of the Stampeders in his era, and he spent many hours at Nick's with his pals. His visit was expected and people who once knew him had gathered to say hello. "He was charming," said Ann Firstbrook, who was with him that day. "He's a great actor. He pretended he knew them."

One of the men who sat with him for a while that evening in Nick's was a former Calgary quarterback and for a time Terry's roommate on the road. Terry could not recollect ever seeing him before. "You used to break curfew," he told Terry, with a grin, "and you never took me with you."

Terry grinned back. "Those were great times," he said, a neat evasion.

The curious aspect of Terry's amnesia is that he can remember such places as backyards and Nick's, but he can't populate them. When visiting a location he once knew, he sometimes recognizes it, but in his memory it is empty of life. His own understanding of this peculiarity is that he lost all memories with an emotional content.

That's also what neuropsychologists think happened. What Terry is missing is episodic memory, people's storyline about themselves, also known as autobiographical or personal memory. This is overarched by what some believe to be the umbrella of the system, autonoetic consciousness, the term given the splendid continuity that enables everyone to glide mentally between a reminiscence and a plan for next week's outing while dicing onions. This depends on familiarity with oneself. People who know themselves thoroughly can travel effortlessly in time. It is now believed by many neuroscientists that the brain's left prefrontal cortex absorbs experiences and then classifies them for delivery to appropriate storage points elsewhere. The function of the right prefrontal cortex is to retrieve the material that the left prefrontal cortex has sent off for storage, so that autonoetic consciousness gives wings to thought.

When people want to reflect on a recent error of judgement and picture themselves handling the situation better in the future, their right prefrontal cortex finds and assembles information scattered all over the brain to allow review of behaviour in similar circumstances and reflection on the various outcomes. The same area, the seat of such wisdom as the human possesses, then considers alternatives and informs the brain to shape up next time with a better reaction.

The kind of memory that goes with episodic memory is semantic memory. This is a separate system dedicated specifically to facts and objects, and mainly devoid of emotional associations. The ability to know that coffee is a brown powder lies in semantic memory; the ability to make coffee is in a different place, described as procedural memory. Terry's recognition of his Jeep is a semantic memory; his ability to drive it comes from implicit or procedural memory, which sometimes doesn't seem to involve the hippocampus at all. It is the kind of memory people employ when they tie shoelaces without thinking about what they are doing.

But Terry couldn't remember how to shave himself. However, he got into his Jeep and backed it out of the parking space first try. *How come?* A different storage bin.

People can call back from one location in the brain the look of their childhood home, which lies in their semantic memory, but the memory of people who lived there is in another, usually interactive, place, the episodic memory. The process of blending the two is effortless and much of it, like most brain activity, happens at the unconscious level. The resultant composite is rich in sounds, sights, and feeling, all of them recruited from different places in the brain. Without the episodic piece of the memory, what one gets is Terry's empty house.

Terry's episodic memory remains beyond reach. All the settings he has retrieved from his past are lifeless. For instance, Terry has a flash of memory of his childhood bedroom crowded with beds. His mother told him his room held three or four bunk beds for himself and his brothers. He can picture that, but his recall doesn't include the sounds, smells, or sight of his brothers and himself dressing in the congested space. He has no idea if he slept in a top bunk or a bottom one, though placement is a matter of great importance for children and there must have been struggles over territory. The strains of sibling conflict have vanished, along with memories of his siblings, some of whom he would not recognize on the street.

After his injury he readily could identify a football or his golf clubs (semantic memory), but he didn't remember playing either game (episodic memory).

Experiences involving intense emotion remain with most people forever and sometimes are referred to as "flashbulb" memories. Terry's feelings at his father's funeral are gone, however, despite his deep grief that day, and so is his joy at Tracy Lee's birth – which he witnessed – and the hurt he felt that morning the Argonauts fired him without pity.

When someone tells him about a crazy prank they pulled together thirty years ago, Terry can get a piece of it. Something about the story has a familiar ring and he laughs with genuine pleasure, though he can't contribute anything. He can't place himself in the story and can't make a picture of it in his mind, but he *feels* that it truly did happen. "That's great," he will say sincerely. "We had a wonderful time."

Once Terry had a visit from some men with whom he had played baseball as a kid in Pointe St-Charles. They told him he had been the catcher, and sometimes pitcher. That registered. He somehow *knew* he had been a catcher and pitcher. They said that no one ever stole home when he was at the plate because they knew he would run them over. He laughed about that; it sounded just the way he expected he had played ball.

Despite the carnage, music can sometimes stir his memory. Once, driving with Jennifer and listening to the radio, he said, "Hey! That's Boney M. *Yes*, that's Boney M." Jennifer couldn't believe it. "It *was* Boney M," she said, shaking her head. "How did he do that? And he also recognized Paul McCartney. It's amazing."

The music centres of the human brain, oddly enough, are durable constructs that are laid down somewhere in the middle months of fetal development. Evidence abounds that six-month fetuses can hear and remember their mother's songs. The permanence of musical memory causes people to marvel at themselves.

People can recall tunes and lyrics of hits from their teens. Elders are perplexed every now and then when, out of the blue, the song in their heads is one they haven't heard for fifty years and forgot they knew.

The brain also protects its memories of smells. The sense of smell evolved early because being able to discern scent was a necessary skill for early humans to track prey. The capacity is almost latent in modern humans but adults who lose their sight rapidly develop a keen sense of smell that is closer to that possessed by their ancestors. It is a peculiarity of the brain that smells are highly evocative triggers to old memories. The pungent aromas of a forest or kitchen immediately conjure up memories of walking in the woods with friends or coming home for dinner, and a perfume brings to mind the person who wore it.

Both smells and sounds stir memories and reflection, but not for Terry. His thoughts can't drift and when he tries to direct them, the content is thin. For instance, he says he likes to think about his father. What goes through his mind? "His strength . . ." he explains, his face lighting up. "The big family he raised well though he had little background. That he did everything humanly possible as a father to provide shoes and food, and individual care and understanding. He wanted us to be tough." That's true of John Evanshen but not the whole truth. Having no memory of his father, Terry has the unusual luxury, not available to any but those far gone in denial, of imagining that his parent was perfect. In his version, John Evanshen was not a feckless rascal and never frightened his sons with his terrible wrath. In fact, Terry doesn't visualize a corporeal John Evanshen at all, because he cannot form a mental image of his father. When he wants to think about him, he can only review what his family has told him. When he wants to picture him, he checks a photograph hanging in his front hall.

However, Terry does know where the photograph is located. His brain in recent years has been able to store a wealth of well-practised routines. Through the wonders of repetition, new pathways have been worn to permit him to access those memories he needs to carry out habitual tasks. He has no trouble driving himself from the farm to Pearson airport and leaving the Jeep in a park-and-fly when he needs to take a plane. He finds his way to his health club with no difficulty. If he decides to buy new socks, he knows exactly where he can find what he wants.

His new memories, however, are composed primarily of such operational matters and do not much concern themselves with people. He can think about repairs to his car, or the zoning restrictions on his farm, or the state of his wardrobe, but if he encounters someone who has a new baby, he won't remember he knew about the birth unless the person starts to talk about the child. Then many details about the birth come into his consciousness and he can chat about it knowledgeably. Without such prompts, his storage–retrieval system seems confined mostly to his semantic memory system, the category of factual matter.

Terry's memory for one-time occurrences is elusive. One day in the spring of 1999 he returned from giving a successful speech in Regina, elated that it had gone very well and the audience accorded him a standing ovation. He talked about it the next day, still warmly pleased with his reception, and he had stories to tell of what people did and said. He was asked if he would still remember in two days.

He hesitated, weighing the question. "If you remind me that Regina was terrific," he said carefully, "I'll remember it. The picture comes back again. It's as though the electrodes are misfiring and all of a sudden they connect again." In two weeks? A longer pause. "You'll have to tell me the whole thing," he confessed, "and then I'll recognize that it happened. Otherwise, it's gone."

Even eleven years after the accident, Terry's brain can do no better than that. Asked what he did yesterday, he always has to stop and think. Often nothing comes to mind, except that he probably went to the gym and cleaned the barn. If someone says, "You played golf with Don," it clicks at once. He *did* play golf with Don McIntyre. And he had a few good holes. He might even tell you about his drive on the fifth hole.

The accepted wisdom is that memory is stored in designated "bins" all over the brain. The memory people summon up of a birthday party is assembled from the separate places where RNA/DNA molecules containing pieces of our memories of visuals, smells, sounds, and feelings are scattered. An effort to recall an afternoon in Lisbon ten years ago requires neurons strewn in widely spaced locations to fire up and collaborate in a flash. Scientists were awed when they first realized that the brain stores memories of smells in one location, visual memories in another, memories of sounds somewhere else. Something has to alert all these separate locations to spin their Rolodexes and find the matching coded pieces that combine to make a complex whole memory. One of these days, scientists will know how that trick is performed, but right now they can only marvel.

The key to long-term storage in a healthy brain is interest and concentration. Information that people need or want to retain makes it into long-term memory by an act of will. The brain seems to register new information best when there has been a conscious decision to remember it, as when birders fix in their minds the markings of a lark bunting. Also, situations that evoke intense emotion imprint themselves vividly and effortlessly. At deaths and delights, the brain slams itself into its maximum performance, neurons firing in every direction, and the record usually is permanent.

Distraction, however, interrupts the serious work of registering a memory. Few people can hold a phone number in their heads when someone interrupts them between looking up the number and beginning to make the call. People going into another room to get scissors will stare around helplessly, wondering why they went there, if something captures their attention en route.

In *Memory and Amnesia*, Alan J. Parkin, professor of experimental psychology at the University of Sussex, explains that memory is the confluence of two main functions of brain power: storage of information and maintenance of a retrieval system. Even people with alert, well-trained brains, however, do not remember everything that has ever happened to them, although in the 1940s the brilliant Montreal neurosurgeon Wilder Penfield thought so. When Penfield was performing his astonishing brain surgery, opening up skulls with an air-driven chisel and tickling the brain of fully conscious people, he came to believe, and persuaded others in his field to agree, that people retain memories of everything that happens to them starting from birth. He declared that the only reason people can't recall absolutely everything is not because the memories haven't been stored somewhere, but because the brain's retrieval system is inadequate to the task of finding them.

Scientists now are convinced that the brain can't be bothered storing everything, but operates on the garbage-in, garbage-out principle. Most of what people experience is remembered only briefly. Mundane activities of no special significance leave no trail, especially as people age. The best memory machines in the world exist in children, who are avid for information and soak up an amazing amount of material, including trivia, with such intense concentration that much of it makes a permanent imprint. The smells and sounds of youth are so indelible that even very old people can summon up lengthy stories from their childhoods. As brains age they either become less interested in retaining the memory of events or less capable of interest in them, so that days slip by, unrecorded. If old people choose to write their auto-biographies, as an increasing number of them are doing, the first half of the book might take them to age twelve. After that, things speed up.

Despite some people's insistence that they can remember being born, neuropsychologists believe that babies and toddlers cannot store event memories to any significant degree. They are not amnesic, in the true sense. Infants are highly impressionable at the emotional level, and their cognitive development is proceeding at a breathtaking pace. It is simply that their tape recorders for scenes haven't yet developed. At four months, babies will be interested in seeing themselves in a mirror but they don't associate the small person they study with themselves. At eight months, providing the environment is benign, they are becoming thinking entities who can make choices based on the small body of experience they are assembling. Between the age of two and three, toddlers will remember happy times and frightening ones. Around age four, children develop self-awareness and their brains are beginning to function almost as adults' do. The pace of the long learning process that lies ahead begins to slow. The brain has laid down the wiring that will influence adult behaviour forever. Without making a sound or leaving a trace.

In those places and times in human history when written language was either unknown or not much available, the society's most treasured people were those with the best memories, since they were carriers of the tribal legends. Memory training was probably practised all over the world – in modern Kyrgyzstan, which lies between China and Russia, memorization keeps alive the tiny nation's cultural history, which is largely unwritten but has been preserved for centuries by recitation, even though it is contained in a poem of more than a half million lines.

It was the ancient Greeks who first made an art of memorization and gave it the modern name, mnemonics, from Mnemosyne, the mother of the Muses. The method employed by the Greeks was passed on to the Romans and turned up afterwards in European culture in the Middle Ages and among the Victorians, for whom reciting from memory was after-dinner entertainment. In order to learn a long speech, Greek orators first envisioned a room crowded with objects. They pictured the door and then committed the first few paragraphs to memory. The next paragraphs were attached to the bench on the right of the door, and the next to the window beside it. By walking into the imaginary room and around it, the speech would emerge, chunk by chunk, from their memory.

By this means, the historian Frances A. Yates writes in *The Art of Memory*, Seneca the Elder could repeat two thousand names in the order they were given to him. Augustine had a friend who could recite Virgil backwards. Thomas Aquinas developed such perfect recall that as a boy he could recite back everything his teachers had said.

As recently as this century, North American schools insisted that children commit to memory long passages from Shakespeare's plays and a good deal of nineteenth-century poetry. Most white-haired Canadians can still quote Lady Macbeth's speech about the dagger and the first verses of Keats's *Endymion* – "A thing of beauty is a joy forever . . ." In the stimulus-starved prison camps of the Second World War, men with prodigious memories were teachers around whom others clustered.

As brains grow old, they are sluggish when required to yield the name of a familiar person who is approaching. What many people do in such emergencies is employ an adaptation of Grecian mnemonics. They recite the alphabet in their heads, looking for an associative link: A, B, C, *D*! David, Douglas, Duncan . . . *Don*. The well-worn "Thirty days hath September . . ." is still the way most people remind themselves how many days are in the months, another mnemonic.

Similarly, when people are in an unfamiliar neighbourhood, they keep their bearings by means of mental snapshots. The first snapshot is in the parking garage, where a picture of the car's location is taken. Down the elevator and out on the street. Note the name of the street. Turn right at the fruit stand. Straight ahead to the bank, turn left to the destination. The person never gives a thought to any of this while conducting whatever business made the trip necessary but on the return trip the photographs spill out in proper order: right turn at the bank, straight to the fruit stand, turn left, parking garage, elevator to the second floor, and there is the car.

While the world waits for a breakthrough that might provide an understanding of how memory works, some of the prevailing research seems odd to a layperson. For instance, some scientists are trying to identify which foods most benefit memory, starting from the observable truth that diet plays a role in brain function. As teachers well know, malnourished children have more difficulty learning than do nourished children. Famine, such as that experienced in Africa and North Korea, does permanent damage to children's brain development.

It was established early in this line of inquiry that glucose, a common sugar, stimulates brain activity. In 1999, Randall Kaplan, a post-graduate student at the University of Toronto, conceived of a small but intriguing study which found that aged people with slowing brains perked up temporarily fifteen minutes after eating mashed potatoes or barley, which seem to stimulate their acetylcholine, one of the brain's neurotransmitters. And people who run or do other vigorous physical activities are stimulating their brain power, probably because exercise boosts cardiovascular systems and stimulates the production of endorphins.

Terry's brain can't make the information available to him without a great deal of repetition, or "overlearning," as neuropsychologists call it. When healthy brains are put to the same task over and over, they will alter themselves so the task can be done without conscious thought. Structural change happens when people use a pathway inordinately. The synapses needed to accomplish the new task grow stronger, while the ones in disuse weaken, and a highway is created. For instance, sighted people have far less ability to interpret sensation in their fingertips than do in people who read Braille, because the latter overuse that part of their brains.

Accordingly, if people addicted to a certain unwanted behaviour wish to discourage their brains from compelling them in that direction, they have only to desist from the behaviour for a period of time. Nail-biters who consistently deny the impulse to chew on their cuticles eventually will stop feeling the urge each time they are anxious; the brain forgets.

Terry misses his past, sometimes acutely, but he is grateful that he can't remember the accident at all. "I would hate to relive that in my dreams," he says.

Ten years after the accident, he started to dream again. This interests neuroscientists because studies of where dreams lurk in the brain now seem to indicate that damage to frontal lobes will cause the injured person to stop dreaming. Dr. Mark Solms, a neuropsychologist and psychoanalyst in London, England, has been studying dream cessation for almost twenty years and concludes that the forebrain has to be part of a relay system. If that is true, Terry's frontal lobes are making new links.

Terry's dreams, however, are colourless and dehumanized, and empty of emotion, the characteristic of semantic memory. His dreams are about household matters: the trivia of errands and chores. He doesn't see people in his dreams.

Minute change has been happening steadily. Terry's unrelenting efforts to observe the rules of politeness and consideration are bearing fruit. He has learned the rules of social behaviour. He gradually is putting together a sociable personality who welcomes guests, makes introductions, and offers coffee. These gains are all the product of overlearning. With Lorraine's coaching over many years, civility is becoming instinctive in him. He expresses concern when he hears about someone's flu, and he pays compliments when he receives a gift. Lorraine, even when she is most impatient with him, concedes that he is becoming a nicer person.

What hasn't changed, as yet, is Terry's inability to initiate a conversational topic, though he can follow and contribute appropriately to whatever topic someone else launches. He doesn't read faces or body language well enough to know how others are feeling. He can't sense a mood change in a room in order to adjust his behaviour.

A small but significant incident occurred in December 1999, when Terry was confronted with a choice he had to make — whether to accept a sponsor's suggestion that he stay in town an extra day on a weekend in order to qualify for reduced air fare. Terry was inclined to agree but Lorraine was opposed. He wakened the next morning with his mind made up: he would not stay the extra day.

He was surprised at himself. He doesn't know where that decision came from, except that his brain must have been working on the problem in his sleep.

Many people have had the experience of waking with the solution to a concern that was vexing them when they went to bed. It now is known that brains are hives of industry while people sleep. When examined with electrode tracers, they light up all over the place with activity that might relate to filing data or might be minor circuit repair. Apparently, while asleep, brains can continue a line of thought that was active when the person dropped off. What is interesting in Terry's case was that this was the first time in his post-accident life it had happened to him. It was so unusual that he thought for a while it must have been a dream. However it was done, it signified that somewhere in the executive part of his brain, where decisions are made, a skill for future-planning was reviving.

Neuroscientists doubt very much that Terry will ever achieve much more than incremental gains. Their educated guess is that memories of his life before the accident will never return, and they don't hold out much hope that his short-term memory will improve a great deal more than it has. The most blighting expectation is that Terry will always be emotionally somewhat flat: kindness and empathy are hard for an adult to grow from scratch. In an experimental daycare setting at the Hospital for Sick Children in Toronto a few decades ago, two-year-olds lacking empathy because of rough early experiences could be taught to think of others, but three-year-olds were much more hardened.

Nor are the experts optimistic that Terry will ever regain the spontaneous warmth and affection he once exhibited, or ever fully be able to control his terrible temper. But they confess that they simply cannot be sure. Tools such as the imaging technologies that show changes in the brain are only a few years old. Subjects with injured brains are being followed to see what develops, though research money for this is scarce, but not enough time has passed for any conclusions to emerge.

"Each person is individual in how they recover," Don Stuss, neuropsychologist, says. "We are finding people recovering cognitive abilities ten, fifteen years after the injury. We used to believe that never happened. So something seems to recover on a long basis. Does empathy recover? We don't know."

Terry's steady progress brings all glum predictions into question. The Evanshens see Terry getting better and they cling to the hope that Terry is on a path of steady and continuous improvement. He believes with all his heart that he is a good man and becoming a better one every passing day. And he won't quit. That's just not in his nature, brain damaged or not.

ELEVEN

Tracy Lee Evanshen was married to Joseph Clark on September 14, 1996, and a drenching rain fell on the Evanshen farm as the reception began in a fortuitously rented white marquee in the apple orchard. The bride's sisters, Tara and Jennifer, were lovely in floor-length burgundy gowns with long white gloves and sprays of calla lilies on their arms. Joseph, a tall and astonishingly good-looking young man who aspires to be an actor, wore a well-fitting tuxedo, as did the bride's father. Terry's face radiated joy and confidence, though he could recognize only a few of the almost two hundred guests, and Lorraine's beaming smile in the wedding photos is belied by the fatigue in her eyes. This was not a family like other families, and the wedding preparations had taken their toll on all of them, especially Lorraine.

When Terry speaks of the wedding, what he remembers first is that four of the guests were in the Canadian Football League Hall of Fame, not counting himself, and that many others were former football players or coaches from the four CFL teams on which he played. Their presence was testament to the affection and loyalty the scrappy man inspired in his teammates, and he is appreciative.

The rest of his family can't think of the wedding without remembering the pre-marital uproar. The acrimony leading up to the event was so bitter that Tracy almost fired her sister Tara as a bridesmaid. Tara was stuck for weeks in a towering rage over the exclusion from the guest list of her boyfriend, Ray Lazenby. That edict came from Terry, and Lorraine agreed with him. Lazenby, a young man with a gleam in his eye who later, at twenty-two, fathered a child, perhaps reminded Terry in some subliminal way of the wild youths he had known in Pointe St-Charles. Whatever the reason, Terry's ban of Lazenby turned Tara into "ten miles of rough road," as a family friend put it. Tara explains the dispute laconically, "My dad and I are both set in our ways. We both want to be right all the time."

Tracy had a moment of sadness on that happy day, but not about her stunning but tumultuous sister. In a reflective moment as she watched her father laughing with her new husband she thought wistfully, "Dad has known Joe as long as he's known me. He met us both for the first time after the accident."

Following the beautiful wedding, the Evanshens suffered a serious of brutal blows that fell with the force of a hammer on an anvil. The first occurred on March 17, 1998, when the family was in Aruba for its annual vacation. Tara got word that morning that Ray Lazenby, her love, had been stabbed to death outside an Oshawa bar in the small hours of the morning. Their relationship had ended for a while over his affair that produced a child, but the couple had been reconciled for some time.

Tara was home in time for the funeral. Because her parents had disapproved of Lazenby, it was difficult for them to offer her the unencumbered comfort she needed. She went instead to Lazenby's parents, their shared grief drawing them together. For a young woman, only twenty-two, it was an overwhelming loss. "I keep my depression to myself," she says. "I think I had maybe a mental breakdown for a while. But then I decided there had to be a reason why these things happen. There's got to be a reason."

Tara had an urge to leave home but she had no particular skills and most of her jobs after she quit college were of the casual, dead-end variety. She was thinking of applying to work on a cruise ship or maybe joining the army, when the second blow to the Evanshen family fell and tore out their hearts.

It began innocuously. In 1996, soon after Jennifer turned eighteen, she started to have the occasional intense headache. Jen had never been known to have headaches at all, and these were beauts that came in clusters, with intervals of five or six months without a headache at all. Once, she was in such pain, she missed two weeks of college. The next summer, the headaches grew worse. The Evanshen family doctor told her she was having severe migraines and prescribed medication, which didn't work.

Tara was not convinced that her sister's headaches were only a nuisance to be endured with the family's trademark stoicism. Tara listened to Jennifer throwing up non-stop at night in the bathroom, and checked Jen's symptoms with people who had a diagnosis of migraine headaches. Their experiences and Jen's didn't match.

"I think she's got a tumour," Tara said insistently to the family. "You have to check it out." At first Terry and Lorraine dismissed Tara's fears, but when Jennifer started to have difficulty seeing objects on her right side they took her to Doug Waller, the neurologist. Waller could find nothing to suggest that Jennifer had anything more than migraines and prescribed some migraine medication. "Come back if she doesn't get better," he advised them.

In August, Jennifer woke up one morning with bloodshot eyes. She bought eye drops, but they were ineffective. The redness, in fact, was a brilliant, even colour that looked as though her eyeballs had been painted. The people at her summer job stared at her in consternation.

In the fall, the headaches were so immobilizing that Jennifer was not able to attend the first week of classes at the college where she was to begin her third year in a hospitality training program. On September 8, 1998, her twenty-first birthday, she forced herself to drive to the college but could not stay for the pain. On the way back to the farm the right side of her body went numb, as if she had had a stroke. Driving with one hand, she got home and told her mother something was wrong.

Terry drove Jennifer to the Oshawa General Hospital emergency room and asked for Doug Waller. Though he was not on call, Waller came at once. He found her reflexes were fine, but there was one symptom, a slight blurring, that seemed out-of-the-ordinary for migraines. Though symptoms of serious trouble were absent, he had a hunch that something was very wrong. "Intuition is unconscious logic," he comments tersely. He arranged for a CT scan, and when he saw the printout he ordered an MRI, which was done at dawn the next morning instead of the usual wait of months. He studied the results in horror, but kept what he saw and his feelings to himself. Jennifer appeared to have an extensive growth on her brain. "There's something I don't like about this," he told Jennifer calmly. "I think we'll do another scan." The next

MRI was the same. Waller contacted a neurosurgeon at Toronto's St. Michael's Hospital and asked him to assess the tests. Jennifer was shocked that Waller wanted her to pack a bag and check in at once at St. Michael's.

After an unsettling three-hour wait in the hospital emergency room, a young doctor told her that a "little lesion" had been found on Jennifer's brain and she would be admitted. After a few days of hanging around her hospital room, her apprehension growing, Jennifer, still in her hospital gown and slippers, was taken by taxi to Wellesley Hospital for a biopsy of the "little lesion." When it was done she returned to St. Mike's, where she was discharged and told to return in a week.

The neurosurgeon she was scheduled to see in a week decided to give her the results of the biopsy and brain scans over the telephone instead of waiting for the appointment. His behaviour is difficult to condone. "You have a tumour," he told Jennifer on the phone, "and it is not benign. The good news is that it is the slowest-growing of brain tumours." Jennifer was confused. Things didn't sound too bad, but on the other hand they didn't sound good. And what did "not benign" really mean? The doctor continued, "It's non-operable. It's a little spider-like thing on the left side of your brain. That's why you had the numbness on your right side. Come and see me in six weeks. In the meantime, live your life. Go to school, drive, whatever you have to do."

The Evanshens didn't know what to think. Was it good news that he wasn't going to operate? If it wasn't benign, what was it? Was cancer the only option for "not benign" or was there some other harmless kind of tumour?

Privately Doug Waller deplored his colleague's insensitivity and lack of clarity. "Neurosurgeons are not good at delivering bad news," he explained. "He knew right away that there wasn't anything he could do about it and he didn't like to admit it."

Jennifer was given some medication, including cortisone, to shrink the tumour, and everything seemed fine all through October, except that the cortisone was making her puffy. In November she went to see Doug Waller. "Nothing's really happening," she said. "How about we cut down on my medication?"

"I don't see why not," he replied affably.

A short time afterwards Jennifer had a severe epileptic seizure that terrified Lorraine. The fire and ambulance departments sent rescue units to take the unconscious woman to hospital. "Way to go, Doug," Lorraine told the neurologist dryly. "You really did a great job there."

The cortisone level was restored. Jennifer became chubby and round-faced, which she hated, but the headaches diminished and there were no more seizures.

Waller advised the devastated Evanshens to put their trust in Dr. Norman Laperriere at Toronto's famed Princess Margaret Hospital, one of the major cancer treatment and research hospitals in the world. "He knows those kind of tumours," Waller said. "He knows what works and what doesn't."

Laperriere ordered a sequence of further scans and on December 3, 1998, he advised the Evanshens that the cancerous tumour was spreading. "It has diffused all over your brain," he told Jennifer sorrowfully.

Waller says the cancer invaded Jennifer's glial cells, the housekeeping substance which surrounds neurons to protect them from impurities in the blood. Glia make up about forty percent of brain mass. The tumour had grown over the whole front of Jennifer's brain in the shape of a malevolent butterfly.

Laperriere said, "Think of your tumour as a handful of sand with coffee grains shaken up inside it. What we are going to have to do is get radiation going at a fast clip so we can shrink it as much as possible."

Jennifer pictured herself sick and vomiting after the treatments, her luxuriant blonde hair fallen out, but she kept this distressing image to herself. A week later, when she returned to see Laperriere, he had reacted swiftly to the dire situation. Cutting through a long waiting list for radiation treatment, he had scheduled her to begin that very day an aggressive course of twenty-five treatments: five mornings a week for five weeks.

The family huddled around the kitchen table that night to discuss the logistics of getting Jen to Toronto and back every week day for five weeks. They decided that Terry should be the designated driver, spelled off by Tracy when he was away to give a speech. Tracy was on maternity leave from her job because she was within a month of delivering her first baby.

No one cried. Not in front of the others.

Terry learned the route and where to park the Jeep in the expensive lots that surround the new and beautiful Princess Margaret Hospital in the heart of Toronto. Jen was fitted with a radiation-blocking helmet and mask that exposed only the area of her skull under which the tumour had spread. Though he hates hospitals, day after day Terry waited patiently for hours in the lounge area on the eighteenth floor where pleasant volunteers circulate with drinks and snacks. Terry, his own cognitive difficulties not apparent in this low-key environment, passed the time reading or socializing with the staff and regular volunteers while his beloved youngest child endured radiation that might buy her time.

He was bursting with love and fending off his terror with an act of will because he truly believed that if he ever admitted, even to himself, that Jen was dying, he would undermine her chances of recovery. "She'll be fine," he said to himself like a mantra. "She'll be fine. She'll be fine. She'll be fine."

His advice to Jennifer was cut from the cloth of his own highly disciplined existence. "You have to find something happy to think about every day," he told her with the severe tone he uses when something is important to him. "Don't think about all the bad things. Get your mind focussed on something that is good and concentrate on that."

Ann Firstbrook called almost daily, usually when Terry and Jen were at the hospital, so she could talk to Lorraine and ask how she was managing. During every call, almost without exception, Lorraine was sobbing. Waller's receptionist, Judy Hamilton, observed sadly, "I feel physically sick for Lorraine. This time she's really going to get nailed."

Lorraine was not facing the possibility of a bad outcome. She was saying grimly, "This family has had a miracle before, and we'll have a miracle again."

Tara, close to Jennifer all their lives, had a pragmatic response to the disaster. She said to her sister, "You know you aren't well. I want you to start living your dreams right now." Suffering gave Tara a new perspective on family relationships. Suddenly, her life-long feuds with Tracy were over. One day she blurted out, "Tracy, I really love you." Tracy was transfixed.

Tracy had trouble with the family's refusal to discuss the implications of inoperable brain cancer. "My parents think if Jen knows they are worried, she'll be frightened," she said. "Everyone is being strong and optimistic so she'll be able to do the same. They think if they keep saying she'll be okay, then she'll be fine. I'm different. I'm a firm believer that you have to talk about things, face the reality. We had to face the reality that Dad will never be the dad he was, and we have to face the reality that Jennifer has brain cancer and it's not good."

Still, Tracy deferred to the prevailing strategy of denial. She was touched that Jennifer showed more concern for her sister's advanced pregnancy than she did for her own appalling condition. Whenever Tracy asked how Jennifer was feeling, the valiant reply was, "I'm just fine, thanks. And how are *you?*"

Lorraine noted similarities in the way Jennifer faced her ordeal and how Terry had battled. "Neither of them ever complains," she said. "And Jennifer even has a comedy side to her these days."

During the long drives into Toronto for treatments Terry and Jennifer grew closer than they had ever been. They listened to his favourite tapes, always Rod Stewart, though Jen groaned sound-lessly at the repetition; he was trying to learn the lyrics. They made easy small talk, neither discussing what was most on their minds. Theirs was the companionship of perfect understanding and unspoken love. Whenever Jennifer had meetings with doctors and therapists, she insisted that Terry be allowed to attend. "I want my father with me," she would explain in a level, determined tone not unlike his when his mind is made up. "I want his support."

One day on the drive home Terry could bottle up his feelings no longer. He pulled the Jeep to the shoulder of the road, and said to Jen with tears in his eyes, "Honey, I want you to know that I am proud of you. You are going through this thing with no complaint, and I know you are going to beat it. And I love you very much." He had never been more his former decent, appreciative, kind self. Jennifer thinks that her father found new levels of patience and empathy because of his own familiarity with the grief of brain damage.

Radiation caused Jennifer to lose her thick mane of golden hair in patches, leaving her skull with a large saddle of baldness surrounded by some strands of long hair, almost black at the roots. The effect was odd. Her response was to put on a baseball cap and make a joke of her appearance.

On January 9, 1999, when Camryn Evanshen Clark was born to Tracy and Joseph, Jennifer was almost halfway through her radiation treatments. She was so exhausted after each session that she needed to lie down as soon as she reached home. When she spoke her mind seemed to drift and she mumbled disconnectedly, like her father had in the first few years after his brain injury. Nevertheless, she spent a few hours one evening in her bedroom gathering up her childhood treasures, her favourite stuffed animals, which she gave to Tracy for Camryn. Tracy almost could not bear to take the gift, which felt so much like a farewell.

As the radiation treatments proceeded, Jennifer began to notice problems with her eyesight. Each day, she was having more trouble seeing. She thought that maybe she needed glasses, so she and her father went to see a neuro-ophthalmologist at Prince Margaret. The specialist thought her failing eyesight was being caused by either the medication or the tumour. On investigation, it proved to be the latter. Jennifer's optic nerves were being strangled.

Looking straight ahead, Jennifer could see only grey fog, rimmed all around with a narrow band of vision. In bright light she was truly blind, but in a dim room she could make out large objects. One eye had lost ninety-five percent of its vision and the other eighty-five percent.

The twenty-one-year-old didn't complain, though she admitted missing the ability to read, see television, finish her education, use the computer, drive a car, write a letter, or go to movies. Doctors held out the possibility that her sight would return if her tumour shrank, so she pinned her hopes on that chance. She prayed twice a day in the privacy of her bedroom and started to wear the medal of a protective saint.

On the surface, Terry and Lorraine appeared certain that the blindness was only temporary. "She's young and a very healthy woman," Lorraine said, "so we have to hold on to that. She has a lot on her side."

Lorraine added firmly, "I keep myself very positive. Things are going to work out." Terry, on his part, disliked hearing, even, that something was amiss. Once when Lorraine was explaining about Jennifer's peripheral vision, he interrupted her angrily. "We don't talk like that," he told her. "Stop saying those things."

Lorraine arranged for her niece Lisa Dozois, Clare's daughter and a master plumber, to refit the upstairs bathroom to make it safer and more convenient for Jennifer. An occupational therapist came to show Jen how to orient herself in her room and such potentially dangerous areas of the house as the stairs. A trip to the Canadian National Institute for the Blind was suggested but by common consent was put on hold. Jennifer's sight might return. Besides, the word *blind* represented a kind of surrender.

Jennifer began to have a recurrent dream that she could see. In the dream, she was sitting peacefully on a beach by the ocean, watching the surf roll and break, roll and break. She wakened feeling sad, and said her prayers.

When the radium treatments ended and her strength returned, Jennifer made herself helpful around the house. Every morning she dressed in warm clothes and went out, no matter how bitter the weather, to clean the stalls and tend to the horses. Since the barn was a dim space, she could see well enough to do such rough work.

Early in February, Tara, Jen, and Lorraine were bouncing around the farmhouse kitchen in new clothes and dark tans, the latter obtained in a tanning salon in preparation for the family's annual vacation in Aruba. Lorraine's theory is that pre-tanning protects skin from being burned in the tropical sun. Lorraine's hair, usually ash blonde, was a becoming cap of platinum, and Jennifer had found artful ways to comb her remaining hair over her bald spots. Their merry mood sprang from their unspoken agreement to snap out of their private despair. It would be weeks before Jen was scheduled to have an MRI that would show what the tumour was doing. Meanwhile, the family was learning to live with someone who couldn't see. It was an adjustment to give Jen an answer aloud rather than nodding, but that lesson was behind them. One eye specialist had just said that Jen's sight would never return, another had just said it would. Things were just fine.

Jennifer's MRI took place on March 28, 1999, and Terry drove her to the appointment. That day Lorraine prepared Jen's favourite dinner of roast beef and all the trimmings, including chocolate cake and whipped cream for dessert. The Evanshens were still eating when the phone rang. Lorraine answered and it was Laperriere, Jen's doctor. "I have some good news about the MRI," he said.

Lorraine said instantly, "Jennifer needs to hear this, not me."

Jennifer turned her back on her family as she listened. As they watched she raised her fist in victory, *aw-right!* and then did a thumbs-up. Laperriere was telling her that he was amazed that the tumour had shrunk by a third, a most unusual quick change for what is normally a lethargic tumour. He said he would reduce the dosage of cortisone. Also, he said, Jennifer's eye tests showed no more deterioration. In all likelihood her blindness would not get worse.

Jen, in tears, was hugged by all.

Lorraine said, "Maybe all the nutrients she is taking helped." Jennifer had a large wicker basket, kept on the kitchen table, that was packed with pills Lorraine bought at a health food store. She had learned to grope the lids to identify the contents. "You never know," Lorraine said with a shrug. "You just never know what will make a difference."

Aline, Terry's mother, had a different explanation for the improvement in Jennifer's tumour but she kept it to herself. She feels herself in touch with an Indian spirit world, and especially with one powerful spirit she calls "my friend." She maintains that this connection is largely responsible for Terry's recovery from the accident, and recently she had begun praying confidently for Jennifer's sight to return. "She's totally nuts," sighed one of her grandchildren.

Jennifer's next MRI was on June 17, 1999, but this time Laperriere did not call right away with the results. He even went out of town soon afterwards for his summer vacation without contacting Jennifer with the results. The family refused to let this worry them, at least not aloud, though they were all terrified by the implication that he had bad news that he didn't want to share. When Laperriere returned he had nothing to say about the size of the tumour. Instead he told Jen she was doing just fine and should come and see him again in a few months. No one pressed him for details.

The baby Camryn was a blessing in a family that badly needed something to go right. Terry was besotted with her, a happy and responsive little person, and she with him. He held her lovingly, cradling her in his brawny arms and cooing to her, and she fixed her huge blue eyes on his face with an expression of infant joy. Terry was the one who was best at putting her to sleep, talking softly in her ear as he paced the floor with her snuggled against his chest. Lorraine rolled her expressive eyes. "He'll have her walking by six months," she said wryly. That didn't happen, but when Camryn was only three months old, Terry started to teach her to speak. By six months Terry had spent so much devoted time coaching her that she would say a spluttering, wet "Poppa" when she saw him.

The third Evanshen disaster concerned Aline. Terry's mother and Lorraine had been a good fit, despite their very different personalities. Over the years before and since Lorraine married Terry, their relationship had been pleasant. "Lorraine was more a daughter to Aline than her daughters," a family member said. With the tragedy of Jennifer's brain tumour, however, family tensions sharpened until both Aline and Lorraine began to get on one another's nerves. Aline had been expected to stay in the farmhouse for a year or so and then move on to another relative, but seven years had passed since Lorraine decorated a big upstairs bedroom for her. One of Aline's sons is remote from the family and another is dead, but that still left nine other prospering adult children she could have visited in rotation. But Aline had decided to stay in the farmhouse.

Aline and many of her family seem unaware of the deep damage to Terry's memory that makes life difficult for him and his family. "I don't think they realize the hard work that has gone into Terry's recovery to get where he is today," Lorraine said one day, with Terry in the room. "They don't give him that pat on the back he deserves." Believing Terry to be almost completely himself again, the other Evanshens tend to see Lorraine's close supervision of him as an affront to his male dignity, and evidence that she is a dominating and spouse-withering woman. "Lorraine's people were all bossy, possessive people," Aline said dismissively. For her part, Lorraine – hard-headed about money – didn't think too highly of Aline's compulsion to spend her old age pension on the slot machines at Casino Rama.

Both women coped with the almost untenable situation after Jennifer's diagnosis with as much grace as they could muster. Though Lorraine resented Aline's prolonged status as a pampered house guest, she said nothing to Aline that was rude. Aline was hurt that the family excluded her from confidences, but didn't complain to them. "I go to my room at lot of the time," Aline said, her eyes crackling with indignation. "I don't want to interfere."

By the spring of 1999, Aline's presence had become an irritant that added to the stress the household was undergoing. The older woman was openly critical of Lorraine's protectiveness with Jennifer and she also deplored her daughter-in-law's willingness to let Tara live at home well into adulthood. As Aline pointed out, that was something that didn't happen when her brood reached maturity. Lorraine, whispering despite doors closed to be certain Aline would not hear, had complaints of her own.

Just before Mother's Day in 1999, Aline's son Gordon came to take her home with him to Toronto for a short visit. Aline was happy to go because she finds Gordon easy to get along with. Lorraine took the opportunity to discuss privately with Gordon's wife, Barbara, a plan that had been on her mind a while. Her idea was to find a small apartment, close to public transit, where Aline could live independently. The far-flung Evanshen progeny could chip in to make sure of Aline's continued comfort.

Gordon's wife seemed to think this was a reasonable suggestion, but somehow it lost a lot in transition. The whole Evanshen family, and especially Aline, came to believe that Lorraine wanted to put Aline in a nursing home for indigents. Aline stormed back into the house one day when Terry and Lorraine were out and removed her belongings, leaving behind still-wrapped Mother's Day gifts from her grandchildren. Thereafter she and almost all the Evanshens ceased communication with the family. Terry was devastated, the more so a few weeks later when none of his siblings or his mother acknowledged his fifty-fifth birthday. In the months that followed, there was not a word from his family, not even an inquiry about Jennifer. The exception was Terry's brother Fred, who checked in regularly with Jennifer to ask about her condition.

As the summer of 1999 wore on with silence from all but one of the Evanshens, the strain began to tell on everyone. The bad news that Jennifer's eyesight would never return deepened the gloom that hung over the pretty house. Terry was agitated and depressed, though he denied it. "Terry is an inferno," Ann

Firstbrook said compassionately. "He's having lots of outbursts, more than I have ever seen. It was bad the first year I knew him, but nothing like this." Lorraine was on a perpetual knife-edge to keep herself from weeping or screaming. Tara seemed almost never to be home, and Jennifer – the family's peace-maker – grew more beautiful every day, and thinner, and more quiet. She talked of finding a job, or some useful volunteer work she could do without sight. Weekends she put on short perky dresses, a long blonde wig over the dark and silky stubble that was beginning to grow back, and went dancing with her boyfriend.

Late in the summer, the family got in touch with the Canadian National Institute for the Blind. Jen's new goal was to find gainful employment she could do without much sight.

Her sister Tracy was in despair. "No one talks about the time line," she grumbled. "Does she have five years? Three years? Six months? I don't like what's going on."

The Evanshens that summer were rocked by news that Dr. Doug Waller, the neurologist who had become a close family friend, was charged with sexual assault of a thirteen-year-old boy. Following that, other charges were laid concerning occurrences twenty-five years earlier with older male patients. To its credit, his hospital did not panic. Remembering the man's long history of dedication and compassion, the Lakeridge Health Corporation, formerly the Oshawa General Hospital, issued a statement that Waller would not be suspended because the charges were still unproven.

Lorraine made a phone call to Waller and talked to his shattered nurse, Judy Hamilton, asking that she pass along to Waller her concern. A week or so later, Terry gathered up Jennifer and paid Waller a visit in his office. He put out his hand to the doctor and said, "I'm your friend."

Terry explained, "That man has been wonderful to us. He stood by us all these years. We can't just forget that."

Despite the pressures on him, Terry was loosening up. His speech, while still read off the cards, developed a self-mocking, amused tone when he described his various mishaps. His presentations in the past had been drenched in troubled earnestness, and this new lightness was appreciated. Audience response noticeably improved. In June 1999, Terry received a letter from the chief executive officer of a group in Regina he had addressed a few weeks earlier. The CEO spoke of the "exceptional job" Terry had performed and how Terry "truly touched hearts minds and souls of all of us. You have inspired a cultural change in our organization. . . . You have inspired our people to share . . . This would not have happened prior to your sharing of your story."

Terry gained composure from such encouragement and was finding the confidence in himself to confess to people that he couldn't remember them. When approached by someone who seemed to know him, he no longer bluffed his way through the encounter, letting the other person carry the conversational ball. He was saying without embarrassment, "I'm sorry, but since my accident I have trouble with my memory. If you help me, maybe I'll be able to remember where we met."

That transition took all the willpower he could summon, and came in good part because Lorraine goaded him, telling him over and over to "drop your stupid pride." Terry explained to her that he faked because didn't want to appear ignorant, but she wasn't buying it. To accommodate her insistence, he started an internal argument. "No, they won't think you're stupid if you don't know their names," one Terry would say to the other. "Yes, they will," the other Terry responded. "No, they won't." "*Yes, they will.*" He considered both views in the night when he couldn't sleep, but in the morning he was no further ahead. Finally, however, "No, they won't" won out.

With all the blows that the year had brought the Evanshens, it was no surprise that Lorraine wept easily and started to smoke again, though only outside the house. Her once-saintly tolerance of Terry's peculiarities seemed to be slipping. A typical exchange occurred one lovely summer afternoon when the two were entertaining a visitor in their vast kitchen and talking about Terry's favourite topic, his recovery. The conversation went like this:

Terry, very sure of himself, began with: "I feel I am making progress, so long as I'm going along, being a good person . . ."

Lorraine interrupted coldly, pointedly ignoring him and addressing the visitor: "When you have the kind of injury Terry has had, the kind that has to do with the brain, you become very selfish. Very self-centred. Think of nobody but Terry. To this day I don't feel that Terry understands what quality time is with the family. He's so involved with doing his own thing, whether it is the cutting of the grass or the pruning of the trees. When he's done he's going to sit down, he's going to read, or whatever. Last night was a perfect example. I was sitting in there watching a movie with Jennifer that I watched only because I knew it was going to be downer for her, and I didn't want her watching a downer all by herself. And here was Terry out here in the kitchen reading a paper."

Terry, his face miserable, said, "Honey, please. Listen to me very carefully. The word selfish is not part of my vocabulary, never has been, and is not now and never will be. I am definitely a 'we' person, not an 'I' person. If I ever give that kind of feeling to you or to the family, you must stop me dead in my tracks and say, 'Terry,' quietly, 'you shouldn't do that.' Of course I would need some direction, but my heart is not even one percent selfish. Take that out of your vocabulary. Could you please?"

Lorraine looked away.

Terry said, pleading, "That's not me at all."

The visitor suggested, "That's not who you want to be?"

Lorraine pounced. She said, in a tone drenched with sarcasm, "Yes, that who he *wants* to be."

Terry caught her implied accusation that he wants to be a caring person but really isn't. He could think of nothing in his own defence. Sadness fell on the room as two decent, lonely people sat in dejected silence. What Lorraine really was saying was "I'm scared and exhausted. I need you to show me that you love me, that you love your children." What Terry was trying to convey was, "Please understand, I'm trying my best. I'm lost too."

Lorraine is the first to say, however, that recent years have seen a great improvement in Terry's ability to exhibit tenderness. For a long time after the accident he displayed no sign of concern for others but gradually his artificial hugs became spontaneous and sincerely affectionate. He was very pleased with this development. "The more I practised that hugging, the more I listened to what others were saying, the more I was enjoying it. It's coming back," he said enthusiastically. "I think I am getting empathy now."

Ann Firstbrook, after years of watching the Terry–Lorraine interplay, spoke of their love for one another, which is obvious despite the bickering. "Terry's compulsiveness, his insistence on completing a task no matter how late the hour or unimportant the chore, drives Lorraine nuts," Ann said, "but that's how he functions, that's how he gets through the day. He is constantly frustrated because he expects himself to be perfect. He refers to himself a hundred times a day as an asshole. He is terrified he will slip back, not function even at the level he has now." Lorraine knows that. She has loved Terry since she was a teenager and loves him still, but her terror of losing Jennifer was making it difficult for her to be tolerant of her husband's often irritating behaviour.

Terry admits that even minor frustrations are impossible for him to handle. Lorraine says that one day he opened the hood of the Jeep with such force that he pulled the lever off. "He went ballistic," she says. Soon after that something went wrong with the tractor he was driving and he began to yell again. Lorraine went out to cool him down but she herself was exasperated.

"Terry, this is no big deal," she said indignantly. "You're not going through your whole life without things breaking down. Holy God, get with it."

Jennifer ran out of the house and scolded them both. "I've had it with this arguing the last couple of days," she said. "My parents never used to argue and I'm getting fed up. I'm going to sit down with both of you tonight and you're going to hear a piece of my mind."

Lorraine and Terry grin to remember it. "She was so cute," Terry says fondly.

When Terry lies in his bedroom for his afternoon rest, the thoughts that arise unbidden usually concern his failure to control his temper. He admits freely that he allows minor incidents to expand into major conflicts, and he hates himself for it. The respite time he should spend recuperating his mental resources very often is eaten instead by his bottomless remorse. "I revert back and think, I didn't do that in my first life," he says. "Why am I doing it now? And I start doing it all over again. It is perpetual anguish, every single day. Going over the same things."

A major bone of contention in the Evanshen household in recent years has been the farm. Lorraine was anxious that they sell it, insisting to Terry that it was too big and expensive for them to maintain. Their mortgage now is small and she argued that the million-dollar price it would fetch would allow them to purchase something easier and less expensive to maintain. Terry was adamant that the farm will never be sold. It is, in fact, the only home he has ever known, and he doesn't know how he would occupy himself without the obligation to do barn chores and lawn mowing.

Both Evanshens, raised in poverty and shabby, crowded housing, love living in a handsome residence and deeply appreciate the spacious rooms and vast acreage, but Lorraine places less value on occupying a showplace. She dreams of a compact but private house in nearby Brooklin or maybe a winterized cottage on Golden Lake at Val David. "Something peaceful and quiet," she said wistfully. "Something small. Then maybe Terry would be able to spend more time with me, and not be so tired from chores that he stutters."

Asked why he refused to live in a more convenient, contemporary house, Terry responded sharply, "I don't even think about it. I have enough things on my mental plate to survive every day, to make sure everything around me is all right without having something new to deal with. It would be like climbing Mount Everest every day."

He added, struggling to get his feelings across, "I look forward to coming home to the farm. I look forward to the calmness and serenity and love that is here." Lorraine stared at the ceiling, took a deep breath, and said, "I have a lot of love for him as a husband and father. But sometimes I can't understand what's going through his mind."

The necessity to keep his environment stable has made Terry mulish as well about turning in the Jeep he has been driving since the accident. Its odometer has passed 300,000 klicks and maintenance bills pile up, but from his perspective it is the first car he had ever driven, and his attachment is sentimental. Every inch of it known and dear to him.

What he fears is that adjusting to a strange house or even a strange vehicle will destabilize him and make it more difficult for him to manage his temper. Terry never goes anywhere without repeating in his head, "Keep calm, keep calm, keep calm . . ." He was trained at the Good Samaritan Hospital in Washington to walk away from irritations the moment he feels his anger rising, and he tries to do that, but without notable success. The explosions are brief and quickly forgotten by him, a condition typical of brain-damaged people, but their frequency began to accelerate after the crisis with Jennifer's health. Before that he had reduced his explosions to only one or two a day, but the number rose precipitously after her diagnosis.

In early October, 1999, Terry's anger proved disastrous for his long-standing relationship with Ann Firstbrook. The break came at a speaking engagement in Saskatoon which had several irritating glitches, including a microphone that didn't function and a missing baseball that Terry uses as a prop when he tells the story of how seeing Nolan Ryan on television turned his life around.

Afterwards there was an unpleasant scene between Ann and Terry.

They returned to Toronto with little more said, but the next day Terry drove to Ann's house and said he was making a change. He asked her for the name and phone number of a speakers' bureau, Speakers' Spotlight, which Ann had mentioned several times as being willing to work with him when the time came for her to go. Then he left abruptly.

Ann was happy to be finished with travelling with Terry because she had been longing to have more time for her son, Andrew, who was now a two-year-old with tantrums of his own. She had been looking for a propitious moment when she could turn Terry over to the agency she had chosen but she had delayed doing so because of the uncertainty about Jennifer's health. "I just didn't see myself for the rest of my life as a person whose primary responsibility was to keep a fifty-five-year-old man from blowing his top," she explains ruefully. "But I didn't expect it to end this way."

After five years of a very close relationship with the Evanshens, the suddenness and bad feelings surrounding the break came as a crushing blow to her pride. She feared that their friendship had ended as well, but this concern proved groundless. Terry, in a cheery mood, called a week later to ask how she was doing, and how Andrew was. The two began meeting for coffee from time to time and Terry came by at Christmas with a wagon full of blocks for Andrew and champagne for Ann and John.

A few days after the break with Ann, Terry was in an exuberant mood as he described his new relationship with a young couple, Martin and Farah Perelmuter, who run Speakers' Spotlight. "I'm on a new plateau," he explained, beaming. "I'm going to be travelling by myself, but I am ready for that."

A month or so later he went to Vancouver for his first un-escorted speaking engagement. Lorraine saw him off with the reminder to be good, "like sending a kid off to school the first day," she smiles. Terry dutifully recited to himself, all the way to Vancouver, "Be calm. Be calm. Be calm."

The trip was uneventful and he was met in the Vancouver air-port and driven to his hotel without incident. Just before the speech he checked on the VCR equipment he would need and tested the microphone. He is experienced in this technology and calmly asked for adjustments. The speech went well and he returned home in triumph, assuring his wife that he had not blown up even once.

The Perelmuters subsequently devised for Terry a check list, headed "Presentation Details," which each Evanshen sponsor fills in. It leads off with the title of the event and its location, Terry's airplane arrival time, the name of the person who will meet him at the airport if this applies, the name and address of the hotel, the name of the person who will have responsibility for the baseball and video he uses in his presentation, provision for a microphone test about an hour before the speech, and so on, to the time of his departure. With this in hand, Terry confidently embarked on a heavier speaking schedule than he had ever known and was able to travel alone.

A striking aspect of the Evanshen household that last summer of the century, which the separation from Ann Firstbrook accented, was how isolated Terry and Lorraine were. Though Terry and Lorraine appear gregarious, they have withdrawn from most of their friends. Barry Brown, the family therapist who came to know them well, observed that Terry avoided social occa-sions because of his fear of embarrassing himself, and Lorraine had dropped her former busy social life because Terry's behaviour was so unpredictable. The result was, as Brown noted, that the couple lived in seclusion.

The slide into solitude began soon after the accident. In January 1990, Toronto psychologist Dr. George R. Wilkinson noticed Terry's "diminished need for friends." Terry and Lorraine know many people who value them highly but they see them almost never. Tara explains that her father's emotional instability makes reciprocal dinner parties, the common currency of social exchange, out of the question. For her own social life, Tara tries not to have her friends visit the house. When this cannot be avoided she either prepares them to accept that Terry won't remember them or else she coaches her father just before their arrival so that he might fix their identities in his mind.

She finds it stressful, either way. "It's just easier not to have people come here," she says with a shrug.

Occasionally Brian Murray phones Terry from North Bay. He's a school friend from Pointe St-Charles. He and Terry were never close because Murray is a few years older, which seems an unbridgeable gap to teenagers, but they shared a keen interest in football. "It was a rough, tough place in those days," Murray reflected fondly. "Terry is still the same guy today that he was then, kind of quiet and very determined."

He adds, "Terry and Lorraine don't seem to have a lot of friends coming around. They are pretty private, I guess, so I just pick up the phone every now and then to say Hi. Terry's an inspiration to me. When things get tough, I just think of him and say to myself, 'We'll get through it.'" Though Terry now remembers who Murray is when he calls, this recognition doesn't happen with friends who don't stay in close touch.

A measure of the couple's isolation is due also to something intrinsic in the Evanshens. The world of poverty and aggression in which they were raised instilled in both a deep suspicion of the motives of others. Terry as a youth "fought from one corner to the next," and, like Lorraine, remains wary of those who would patronize or criticize him. Unless their intuitions tell them that they are dealing with open and honourable intent, their normal expectation is that others are out to take advantage of them. Both are guided strongly by their instincts about people and the word "trust" comes up frequently in their conversations. People are not good or bad; they are trusted or not trusted.

When the Evanshens trust someone, they are extraordinarily generous, loading visitors with gifts of farm produce, baked goods, and flowers. When they don't believe in someone's sincerity, they turn to ice. "If I don't like you, you don't want to meet me in an alley," Terry once said.

In November 1999, the esteemed television personality Pamela Wallin invited Terry to be a guest on her half-hour interview show. Terry looked his best, buffed to a bronze gleam, and gave the country a portrait of a severely brain-damaged but game man. Her opening questions, "How do you begin to create a human being?" and "How do you know who you are?" were outside his scope. He answered anyway, eager to please and touching in his earnestness as he floundered through disconnected and seemingly irrelevant praise of Lorraine. What he meant to say, and thought he was saying, was that Lorraine had taught him who he had been, and that's how he constructed the approximation he has become.

One of the ways the Evanshens comforted themselves, beginning late that summer, was to take on responsibility three days a week for Camryn. When Tracy finished her maternity leave, Terry and Lorraine agreed to take the baby three days a week, Tuesdays to Thursdays. The stint starts at seven-thirty in the morning and ends about five-thirty when Tracy finishes at the video mail-order outlet in Toronto where she is in charge of assembling the French-language collection. To accommodate their small, good-natured visitor, Lorraine turned what had been Aline's bedroom into a nursery. Terry was ecstatic. He can't get enough of that baby.

Lorraine needed the distraction. The suspense over Jennifer's well-being was making her so distraught that the thought of it would make her weep, which Terry sometimes found irritating. His view was that the family should be satisfied that everything possible was being done, and just get on with their lives. He would say sternly to Lorraine, "And there's always that hope of new medicine, new treatment, and you want to enjoy now the journey, knowing it can and will happen. And if it doesn't . . ." He stopped, then continued, "I want you to keep on that positive note."

Lorraine, her face a mask of misery and tears on her cheeks, would respond from her own solitude, "It's just that she's the one I spend the most time with. I understand her and she understands me . . ." She can't go on.

In January 2000, the family had wonderful news. The results from Jennifer's latest MRI showed continued improvement. Jennifer announced that she needed to work out, and began accompanying her father to the health club every morning. He was delighted. "I know how workouts help me," he says, "and I can see that they are helping her."

He watches out for her. "Don't push it," he warns her fondly.

Terry invented a new mantra for himself. Every morning when he wakens he recites, "You have nothing to complain about. You'll be fine. You'll be fine. *You'll be fine.*"

He really wasn't all that fine. At the end of a long conversation one day, Terry was asked something difficult. What did the man who hit him take away?

He was tired, which meant his thinking process was clogged, and abstract questions always dismay him. He tried to answer anyway. "Oh, I have not even wanted to think that . . ." he began, looking worn and distressed. He started over, "It's not fair for me to think back of who I was and what that guy took away from me. Because then I would really get angry, I think, and, *why me?* and I never want to think like that. That's not my personality. And I just know that the person I am today, I'm touching a lot more people than I did when I played. And so therefore I'm very pleased with what the outcome is."

He paused, getting a grip, and resumed earnestly. "If I've got to do something, let's do a little bit more. If I can give a hundred percent, how about I give a hundred and twenty-five percent? Most people don't do that, but that's them. That's not me . . ." He shifted his position. "You know what? All the pieces that seem to be coming and refolding itself must be a reflection of who I was in the first life. Because so many things now come, and I also know medically that if you are like this you would have a tendency to start to shine like this in your next life."

He knew he was rambling. With an effort, he remembered the question. "The good Lord upstairs allowed me to survive and be productive again, and a good person at the same time," he said quietly. "So I thank him all the time."

ACKNOWLEDGEMENTS

In order to write this book, I spent more than a year with the Evanshens. That family does nothing by halves. I experienced not only their generous hospitality – excellent coffee always waiting when I arrived, and a shower of gifts when I left – but they gave me the matchless gift of their complete trust as I waded into their private lives. I want to thank Lorraine and Terry for that openness and for their friendship, and I am grateful as well to their daughters Tracy, Tara, and Jennifer, for their candour and insights. And thanks also to Aline Evanshen, Terry's mother, who reminds me so much of my own crisp and single-minded French-Canadian mom.

And Clare Dozois, Lorraine's sister, was a delight to meet. I thank as well Terry's football colleagues, J.I. Albrecht, Peter Dalla Riva, and that good person Ronnie Perowne. And also Betty Walker, Don McIntyre, and Brian Murray, friends who shared their reflections with me. I especially thank Terry's long-time agent, Ann Firstbrook, a loyal and wise woman.

The technical stuff in this book was daunting for me because I not only had to describe the complicated trial preparation that followed the accident but also I needed a quick course in the wondrous mysteries of the human brain at a time when neuroscience was exploding with sometimes contradictory discoveries. I was exceedingly nervous of making a mistake. As all journalists discover, sometimes a single missed word or wrong nuance will shatter accuracy. I was privileged therefore to be able to rely on numerous people not only for information but for fact-checking. Whatever errors remain after a considerable amount of due diligence are entirely my fault.

I'll start with the lawyers, Bernie Gluckstein and Fern Silverman, who vetted the legal parts of the book. Paramedics Jim Jack and Andy Benson took me into their world and Jim Jack reviewed the manuscript carefully. The public relations staff at what was once known as the Oshawa General Hospital, Jane DeJong and Eleanor McKay, eased my access immeasurably and with Terry's permission helped me obtain medical files. Emergency-room nurses Marian Timmermans and Angie Bosy were fascinating and informative; Dr. Erik Paidra, emergency-room specialist, was a huge help, and I owe a debt to surgeon Dr. Donald Sproull, who guided me through the events in the operating room and twice checked that part of the book. Respiratory therapist David McKay was a pleasure to meet and I am especially appreciative of the time I spent with Dr. Gary Adams, the chiropractor who helped shape Terry Evanshen's second life.

Thanks too to Barbara Baptiste, a remarkable person and Terry's rehabilitation coordinator; the genial Constable Chuck Nash, who investigated the accident; and neuropsychologist Dr. Ron Kaplan, who works with brain-injured people in his Hamilton clinic. My special gratitude goes to Dr. Catherine Mateer and Dr. Sandra Black, two clinical neuropsychologists at the top of their field, and most especially to Dr. Donald T. Stuss, a neuropsychologist of world renown, and Dr. Doug Waller, Terry's thoughtful and considerate neurologist, both of whom gave me copious amounts of time neither man really could spare, and went over the brain parts of the manuscript more than once.

Michael Levine, who seems to be my agent, got me into this fascinating project, so I want to thank him. Dinah Forbes, McClelland & Stewart's widely respected editor, did a glorious job of spotting redundancies and other mishaps in the manuscript, for which I will be forever grateful. My thanks, too, to Lisan Jutras for her painstaking copyedit. Avie Bennett and Doug Gibson, M&S gurus, were unfailingly supportive and understanding. All rise.

And, finally, my husband of fifty-six years, Trent Frayne, promises to read this book as soon as he has a minute. Meanwhile he continues to steady and comfort and delight me in ways that have made my life glow since I first met him a long time ago in the *Globe and Mail* newsroom. I thank him *a lot*.